C0-CDK-912

Orbital Disease

Orbital Disease
A Practical Approach

Gregory B. Krohel, M.D.
Assistant Professor of Ophthalmology and Neurology
  Albany Medical College of Union University
  Albany, New York

William B. Stewart, M.D.
Director of Ophthalmic Plastic, Reconstructive,
and Orbital Surgery
  Department of Ophthalmology
  Pacific Medical Center
  San Francisco, California

Richard M. Chavis, M.D.
Clinical Assistant Professor
  Department of Ophthalmology
  Georgetown University
  Washington, D.C.

Grune & Stratton
A Subsidiary of Harcourt Brace Jovanovich, Publishers

New York   London   Toronto   Sydney   San Francisco

© 1981 by Grune & Stratton, Inc.
All rights reserved. No part of this publication
may be reproduced or transmitted in any form or
by any means, electronic or mechanical, including
photocopy, recording, or any information storage
and retrieval system, without permission in
writing from the publisher.

Grune & Stratton, Inc.
111 Fifth Avenue
New York, New York 10003

Distributed in the United Kingdom by
Academic Press, Inc. (London) Ltd.
24/28 Oval Road, London NW 1

Library of Congress Catalog Number 81-81529
International Standard Book Number 0-8089-1343-3
Printed in the United States of America

To John E. Wright, M.D., F.R.C.S.,
our teacher and friend.

Contents

optic nerve changes, thickened extraocular muscles, sinus changes, axial length, pitfalls of ultrasound.

Acknowledgments

The authors wish to acknowledge the support of the following organizations and individuals: The Pacific Vision Foundation, San Francisco, California, for their assistance in underwriting the expenses of this book. The National Institutes of Health, National Eye Institute, Bethesda, Maryland, for Training Grant No. EY07037. Research to Prevent Blindness, for an unrestricted grant. Judy Whalen, Lori Dederick, Lisa Neumann, Sonia Simmons, Jenny Houston, and Katherine Snowden, for secretarial assistance. Susy, Ben, and Joe Stewart for their tolerance and encouragement. Judy Tulenko Morley for medical illustrations. David S. Friendly, M.D., Fred Wang, M.D., Steve Simmons, Sughra Raza, Richard Provenzano, M.D., Ivan R. Schwab, M.D., Marc P. Cruciger, M.D., and Bradley N. Lemke, M.D., for reviewing the manuscript.

Foreword

There has long been a need for a book to help the clinician with little experience in orbital disease to examine and investigate patients in a logical and efficient manner. The authors, who are experts in this field, have written a practical guide that should aid the clinician confronted with an orbital problem to take the appropriate steps to reach the correct diagnosis, and subsequently to commence the appropriate treatment.

The general ophthalmologist should have an interest in orbital disease, for the initial management of many orbital conditions is all important. This excellent book will help ophthalmologists to diagnose and treat straightforward orbital problems and to recognize the complications that may necessitate more specialized investigations and treatment than the general clinican might wish to undertake.

John E. Wright, M.D., F.R.C.S.
London, England

Preface

Orbital disease and surgery are emerging as a distinct ophthalmologic discipline. For decades the orbit was under the influence of practitioners primarily involved with its surrounding structures. Ophthalmologists are now actively assuming the role as the primary physicians of orbital disease.

In this book, we provide a clinically oriented, practical approach to the patient with orbital disease. Excellent textbooks are available that are either devoted entirely to the orbit or contain substantial portions concerned with the orbit. These works are often comprehensive and contain superb discussions of orbital disease, usually from the vantage of histopathologic diagnosis. When confronted by a patient with proptosis or other stigmata of orbital disease, the array of signs and symptoms can be overwhelming. The absence of a clinically oriented, practical book based on signs and symptoms of orbital disease, rather than histopathologic diagnosis, has been apparent. We hope we have succeeded in filling this void, and in the process helped to clarify and organize the diagnosis and management of orbital disease.

Gregory B. Krohel, M.D.
William B. Stewart, M.D.
Richard M. Chavis, M.D.

1
History and Physical Examination

The eye, with its complex network of supporting structures, lies within the small, pyramidal-shaped bony orbit. The varied nature of orbital structures within this 35- to 40-cc volume cavity makes possible a wide variety of pathologic processes. In recent years significant technologic advances have improved the diagnostic acumen and surgical expertise of the physicians and surgeons caring for patients with diseases of the orbit. These advances augment but do not replace the thorough clinical evaluation of the patient with an orbital disease process. Clinical skills and the knowledge of the nature of orbital diseases, including signs and symptoms, are paramount.

The small confines of the orbit and anterior location of the eye limit direct observation or palpation of the deep structures. Our diagnostic efforts must be particularly sophisticated as much of what can be learned about orbital processes must be learned through indirect methods.

The history-taking process reveals pertinent clinical facts and allows the physician an opportunity to establish rapport with the patient and patient's family. The history should provide information regarding the characteristics of onset (sudden, gradual), duration (short, long, intermittent), and progression of the disease.

Although a history of proptosis is important, it may not be the chief complaint. Frequently, the patient first reports changes such as decreased visual acuity, double vision, ptosis of the eyelid, tearing, or pain. The development of certain periocular changes in association with proptosis may be very characteristic of specific orbital disorders. For example, variable proptosis that is increased with Valsalva maneuver suggests the presence of orbital varices. The importance of reviewing a patient's old photographs cannot be overstated.

They often provide the best baseline for gauging the development of a progressive orbital abnormality. A complete review of systems and past medical history may alert the examiner to stigmata characteristic of thyroid disease, malignancies, or other systemic manifestations of disease processes that could secondarily affect the orbit.

The examination of the patient with an orbital disease must be methodical and comprehensive. The eye and the orbit are the focus of the physical examination. In addition, the opthalmologist should search for café-au-lait spots, abnormal lymph nodes, thyroid enlargement or nodules, surgical scars, or potential neoplasms in those cases in which orbital findings suggest the presence of systemic involvement. A complete examination of the patient with an orbital disease process may require the consultation of an otolaryngologist, neurologist, neurosurgeon, internist, endocrinologist, and radiologist.

The presence of unilateral exophthalmos implies asymmetry. The possibility of this asymmetry existing on a familial or post-traumatic basis rather than secondary to an orbital mass must not be overlooked.

Exophthalmometry readings may be obtained with a variety of measurement devices. These measurements generally relate the position of the cornea to the lateral bony orbital rims. The measurements obtained on each side are compared to each other and to accepted standards (approximately 14 to 22 mm). They are useful not so much in their absolute value but in assessing the magnitude of asymmetry and in evaluating changes in the degree of proptosis by means of sequential readings. A useful, clinically practical instrument is the Hertel-Krahn exophthalmometer (Fig. 1-1). The proper base width is set to allow the instrument to rest on the anterior aspect of both lateral orbital rims. The examiner may use his or her left eye to examine the patient's right eye, and vice versa. When examining the patient's right eye, the examiner's left eye is open and the patient is asked to look at the examiner's closed right eye. Using the left eye, the examiner aligns the red parallax lines in the mirror. Measurement of the

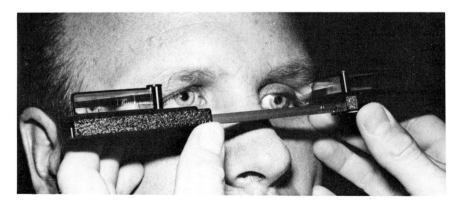

Fig. 1-1. Exophthalmometer in proper position to measure degree of proptosis.

position of the cornea on the mirrored scale is then made. A similar maneuver is carried out for the patient's left eye, using the examiner's open right eye for measurement. Alternatively, the patient may be asked to look at the examiner's forehead with both eyes open while the measurements are made. The technique is not crucial but it must be performed in a similar fashion each time the patient is examined. By recording the base width setting, one can obtain meaningful reproducible measurements for sequential observation.

Proptosis may be axial or nonaxial. Displacement in the vertical and horizontal directions can be measured using a clear plastic ruler, which is positioned horizontally across the bridge of the nose. Both lateral canthi or, alternatively, the medial and lateral canthi on one side, are aligned. Displacement can be measured above and below the plane established by the ruler. Medial and lateral displacement can be measured by making a mark at the center of the bridge of the nose and then measuring the distance from this mark to the nasal aspect of each limbus (Fig. 1-2). As a general rule, the direction of the displacement is opposite to the position of the orbital mass lesion. Anterior lesions, such as fronto-ethmoidal mucoceles (arising medially and superomedially) and lacrimal gland tumors (arising superotemporally) will cause significant downward displacement of the globe in the opposite direction. Posterior orbital lesions, such as intraconal cavernous hemangiomas and meningiomas of the optic nerve, cause a more axial proptosis.

Several other useful physical findings may augment the characterization of proptosis and direct the working diagnosis toward a specific entity. An "S"-

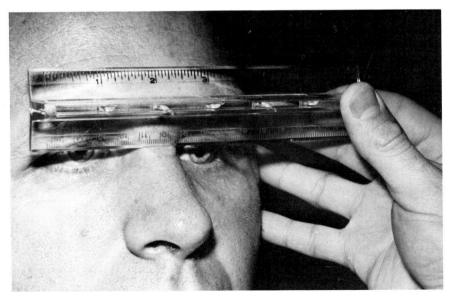

Fig. 1-2. Horizontal and vertical globe displacement measured with a clear ruler.

shaped contour of the upper eyelid, with more prominent swelling laterally, may suggest involvement of the lacrimal gland. Upper eyelid retraction may be a subtle finding, alerting the examiner to the presence of thyroid ophthalmopathy. The presence of lid lag with downgaze will further help substantiate the suspicion of thyroid eye disease. Disturbances of ocular motility may be related to restrictions either caused by mass lesions or secondary to thyroid ophthalmopathy, in which limitation of eye movement is secondary to muscle inflammation. Conjunctival and cutaneous edema and erythema are signs of inflammation and may be seen in thyroid ophthalmopathy, inflammatory pseudotumor, infectious orbital processes, and malignancy. The finding of abnormal periocular vessels should alert the examiner to the potential of vascular anomalies such as arteriovenous communications. Increase of proptosis and/or bluish skin discoloration associated with crying (infant), straining, or Valsalva's maneuver may guide the examiner toward the diagnosis of a vascular abnormality such as an orbital varix. The nasal and oral cavities may harbor readily visualized lesions that have extended to the orbits. The paranasal sinuses and dentition are the most common sites of infections that may spread to the orbit.

Physical examination of the patient with an orbital abnormality must include a complete ocular examination. This examination must include evaluation of corrected visual acuity, pupillary responses, visual fields, and ocular motility. Slit lamp examination, intraocular pressure determination, and dilated fundus examination should accompany the evaluation of the orbit. Intraocular abnormalities such as optic nerve atrophy, opticociliary shunt vessels, chorioretinal striae, or indentation of the globe must be noted. The physical examination should include examination of the conjunctival cul-de-sac and eversion of the lids in search of such characteristic lesions as the anterior, fleshy, salmon-pink lesion of lymphoma.

Palpation may serve only to confirm observed findings or may provide new information about the state of the bony contours and soft tissues. Anterior masses such as lacrimal gland tumors may be easily palpable, whereas masses located more posteriorly in the orbit, whether inside or outside the muscle cone, are rarely palpable. Gentle backward pressure on the globe may cause an anterior prolapse of mass lesions or intraorbital fat. Abnormalities of the bony contours can frequently be readily discerned by palpation. Increased resistance of the orbital soft tissue to retropulsion of the globe suggests the presence of an orbital disease process.

Palpation of the preauricular, submaxillary, and cervical regions for the presence of lymphadenopathy is advisable. Areas of localized tenderness, rubor, fluctuance, induration, or warmth also provide information that may differentiate inflammatory, noninflammatory, and infectious lesions.

The examination of the periocular tissues should include evaluation of the fifth and seventh cranial nerve in addition to those usually studied in a routine ophthalmic examination. A useful test involves careful testing of the sensory branches of the fifth cranial nerve by assessing the response to light touch. Infiltrative lesions such as malignant lacrimal gland tumors may occasionally produce a sensory deficit in the superotemporal region of the eyelid. Most mass lesions displace nerves, however, and do not cause a sensory deficit.

The recognition of orbital pulsation should alert the examiner to the potential presence of an arterially supplied orbital vascular lesion such as an arteriovenous malformation or to the presence of a significant bony orbital defect that is allowing the transmission of cerebral pulsations through the orbit. Orbital pulsation may be noted during gross observation, slit lamp biomicroscopy, tonometry, or in the mirror of the exophthalmometer. Frontal and lateral viewings may be helpful. Observation and palpation for pulsations as well as careful auscultation of the orbits should be part of the complete orbital examination. The laboratory evaluation of patients with pulsations or bruits may include carotid arteriography.

A careful, methodical history and physical examination will lead the physician to a "working" diagnosis. With an appropriate presumptive diagnosis, a pertinent laboratory evaluation can be obtained. The selection of the most fruitful laboratory testing techniques will also depend on a thorough knowledge of the relative prevalence of the most common orbital disease processes. Many series have been published reviewing the prevalence of various orbital conditions. These series, however, vary considerably, depending on whether they review clinical, histopathologic, or radiographic material. Variation is also related to the age of the patients and to the specialty of the reviewer. The most common orbital lesion in children in a histopathologic series may be rhabdomyosarcoma, but neurosurgeons often report optic nerve glioma as the most common orbital mass lesion. Otolaryngologists are likely to report mucocele as the most common orbital tumor in adults, although internists most commonly see thyroid ophthalmopathy. In a clinical series of over 1000 patients seen at the Orbital Clinic of Moorfields Eye Hospital, London, the most common causes of orbital disease were thyroid dysfunction, vascular anomalies, and inflammatory pseudotumors (Table 1-1). Reese tabulated biopsy-proved diagnoses in 504 consecutive cases of expanding lesions of the orbit in adults and children, excluding cases of orbital extensions of retinoblastoma and postirradiation sarcomas (Table 1-2). Two representative series of proptosis occurring in children are listed in Tables 1-3 and 1-4.

In summary, the orbital diseases most frequently encountered in adults by the ophthalmologist are (1) endocrine exophthalmos (thyroid eye disease/thyroid ophthalmopathy); (2) lymphomatous abnormalities (including the spectrum from inflammatory pseudotumor to malignant lymphoma); (3) vascular abnormalities (including the spectrum from orbital varix to cavernous hemangioma), and (4) primary orbital neoplasms. The most frequently encountered orbital diseases in children are (1) orbital cellulitis, (2) dermoid cysts, and (3) vascular abnormalities including orbital varix, capillary hemangioma, and lymphangioma.

Table 1-1
Causes of Orbital Disease in 1041 Patients at Moorfields Eye Hospital*

Thyroid ophthalmopathy	178
Vascular anomalies	148
Pseudotumors	87
Neoplasm (excluding lacrimal gland)	82
Inflammatory	82
ENT problems	69
Fractures and trauma	68
Lacrimal gland tumors	53
Dermoid and other cysts	46
Normal	43
Meningiomas	38
Neurofibromatosis	14
Optic nerve gliomas	13
Neurilemomas	10
Bone changes	10
Others	100

*Wright JW: Personal Communication. Experience at the Orbital Clinic, Moorfields Eye Hospital, City Road, London, England, 1968-1978.

Table 1-2
Diagnosis in 504 Consecutive Cases of Biopsy-Proved
Expanding Orbital Lesions

Diagnosis	Patients (%)
Granuloma (including thyroid ophthalmopathy and pseudotumor)	18
Hemangioma (infantile, 7%; adult, 5%)	12
Lymphoma	10
Lymphangioma	8
Rhabdomyosarcoma	7
Epithelial lacrimal gland neoplasm	5
Neurofibroma, neurilemoma, neuroma	5
Dermoid	5
Mucocele	4
Carcinoma (lid to orbit, 2%; extension, 2%; metastatic, 2%)	6
Malignant melanoma (extraocular spread)	4
Meningioma	3
Optic nerve glioma	2

Data compiled from Reese AB: Expanding lesions of the orbit. Trans Ophthalmol Soc UK 63:85-104, 1971

Table 1-3
Common Diagnosis in 257 Cases of Proptosis

Acute ethmoiditis (orbital cellulitis)
Hyperthyroidism
Orbital hemorrhage (from trauma, leukemia, or scurvy)
Craniostenosis
Hand-Schuller-Christian disease
Cavernous hemangioma
Orbital cellulitis (from trauma)
Orbital cellulitis (idiopathic)
Neuroblastoma
Cavernous sinus thrombosis
Sarcoma
Chloroma
Optic nerve glioma

Modified from Ophthalmic Staff of the Hospital for Sick Children, Toronto: The Eye in Childhood. Chicago, Year Book Medical Publishers, 1967.

Table 1-4
Frequencies of Orbital Tumors in Children

Diagnosis	Patients (%)
Dermoid cyst	29.9
Rhabdomyosarcoma	8.6
Hemangioma	8.0
Lymphangioma	5.7
Optic nerve glioma	5.2
Retinoblastoma	3.4
Neurofibroma	4.0
Inflammatory pseudotumor	3.4
Meningioma	2.9
Microphthalmos with cyst	2.9
Schwannoma	2.3
Lipoma	2.3
Prominent palpebral lobe of lacrimal gland	2.3
Noninflammatory	1.7
Arteriovenous malformation	1.7
Undifferentiated sarcoma	1.7
Teratoma	1.7
Leukemia and lymphoma	1.1
Epibulbar, lid, and orbital osseous choristoma	1.1
Lacrimal gland duct cyst	1.1
Neuroblastoma	0.6
Epithelial or "sebaceous" cysts	0.6
Ectopic lacrimal gland	0.6

Iliff W J, Green W R: Orbital tumors in children, in Jakobiec FA (Ed). Ocular and Adnexal Tumors. Birmingham, Aesculpius, 1978, p. 669

2
The Six P's of
Orbital Clinical Evaluation: Pain

The evaluation of orbital disease is complex and challenging. Our goal is to suggest a useful, methodical clinical approach to diseases of the orbit. The "six Ps" of orbital disease are broad categories labeled by words beginning with the letter "P" that remind us of important aspects in the evaluation of patients with orbital disease. The "six Ps" are pain, progression, proptosis, palpation, pulsation, and periorbital changes.

This method is a familiar technique to all practitioners who have relied on the use of mnemonics and other memory devices throughout medical training. The "seven Ps" of postoperative order writing (i.e., position, pulse, put in, put out, pain, penicillin, procedures) and the "four Ws" of fever workup (i.e., wind, water, walk, wound) were a valuable aid to physicians in training. Hopefully, the "six Ps" of orbital disease will simplify the diagnosis of orbital disease.

Pain and progression represent the patients' symptoms and remind us of the many disease characteristics that should be elicited during the history-taking. Proptosis, palpation, pulsation, and periorbital changes refer to clinical signs sought by the examiner during the physical examination.

Orbital pain, the first "P," must be differentiated from ocular pain and pain referred from the sinuses, nasopharynx, and intracranial structures. The need for a thorough ophthalmologic examination must be emphasized. Dry eye syndrome and convergence insufficiency should always be considered when a routine ophthalmologic exam fails to reveal an obvious cause for pain such as uveitis, keratitis, trichiasis, or angle closure glaucoma. The ophthalmic division of the trigeminal nerve supplies sensory fibers to the globe and surrounding structures and gives rise to distant meningeal branches. Referred pain to the eye and orbit can occur with lesions as far posterior as the occipital cortex. Similarly, the maxillary division of the trigeminal nerve may convey referred pain to the orbit from decayed teeth. Herpes zoster involving the ophthalmic division of the trigeminal nerve can give rise to severe orbital and ocular pain, which may precede the appearance of the characteristic vesicular eruption, which occurs over the periorbital and forehead region.

REFERRED ORBITAL PAIN

Important causes of referred orbital pain are listed in Table 2-1. The most common cause of bilateral retrobulbar pain or aching is the muscular contraction or "tension" headache. Patients usually complain of eye and temple pain in addition to the classic neck and occipital pain. The pain is often worse in the evening and is only partially relieved by analgesics. The headaches can persist for several days. Vision is usually unaffected, and ocular signs are absent.

Patients with the pain of migraine headache often have associated scintillating scotoma and nausea. The pain usually occurs in a hemicranial distribution and usually subsides within one day. There is frequently a history of migraine in the family.

Retrobulbar neuritis produces pain aggravated by eye movement. The pain lasts several days and is associated with clinical signs of optic nerve dysfunction.

Aneurysms of the carotid or posterior communicating arteries can produce intermittent orbital pain lasting from days to years. Diagnosis can be difficult in the absence of a third nerve palsy or other neurologic findings. Fortunately, associated findings indicating intracranial involvement are often present. Carotid occlusive disease will occasionally produce orbital pain. The pain is often aggravated by sitting or standing and alleviated by lying in the prone position. Occlusion of the posterior cerebral artery with occipital thrombosis can cause acute orbital pain which usually lasts one to two days. An homonymous hemianopia on the opposite side supports the diagnosis.

Isolated trigeminal neuralgia involving the ophthalmic division is rare.

Table 2-1
Referred Orbital Pain

Muscular contraction headache
Migraine headache or variant
Retrobulbar neuritis
Ischemic carotid disease
Intracranial aneurysm
Occipital thrombosis
Trigeminal neuralgia
Sinusitis
Dental disease
Cervical disease (arthritis)
Nasopharyngeal carcinoma

Sinusitis will usually be evident on x-ray examination, is often a chronic process, and may be associated with other findings such as localized tenderness over the sinuses and evidence of upper respiratory involvement (e.g., rhinitis). The combination of facial and orbital pain is typical of nasopharyngeal tumors. Cranial nerve palsy and Horner's syndrome are also commonly associated with these insidious tumors. Disorders of lacrimation (dry eye or tearing) and proptosis are less frequently observed. Peak incidence occurs around age 40, and incidence appears to be higher in the Chinese and Maltese. Dental or cervical disease can be best ruled out by physical examination and radiography. The skills of the otolaryngologist, dental surgeon, and neurosurgeon may be necessary in the complete evaluation of patients with orbital pain.

Once satisfied that ocular and referred pain have been ruled out, the clinician can turn his or her attention to orbital lesions. Table 2-2 divides orbital lesions into three categories based on the frequency of accompanying pain.

Table 2-2
Orbital Lesions Categorized by Frequency of Pain

Lesions frequently painful (greater than 75 percent of cases)

    Orbital hemorrhage
    Orbital cellulitis
    Inflammatory orbital pseudotumor
    Posterior scleritis
    Malignant lacrimal gland tumor

Lesions less frequently painful (less than 75 percent of cases)

    Orbital abscess
    Metastatic disease in adults
    Metastatic disease in children
    Phycomycosis
    Osteogenic sarcoma
    Arteriovenous malformations

Lesions infrequently painful (less than 10 percent of cases)

    Sinus mucocele
    Thyroid ophthalmopathy
    Cavernous hemangioma
    Capillary hemangioma
    Varix
    Benign mixed lacrimal gland tumor (pleomorphic adenoma)
    Fibrous histiocytoma
    Dermoid cyst
    Rhabdomyosarcoma
    Lymphoma
    Osseous tumor
    Arachnoidal cyst
    Neurogenic tumor
    Basal cell carcinoma

LESIONS FREQUENTLY PAINFUL

These lesions are painful in more than 75 percent of cases.

Orbital Hemorrhage

The most acute form of orbital pain occurs with orbital hemorrhage, which may be traumatic or spontaneous. The spontaneous hemorrhage presents with the classic triad of sudden pain, proptosis, and nausea or vomiting. In addition, ecchymosis, motility disturbances, choroidal folds, disc edema, and/or visual loss may be seen, especially in the elderly. The underlying etiology is usually an orbital varix (Fig. 2-1). Other etiologies include lymphangioma, blood dyscrasia, hypertension, and anemia.

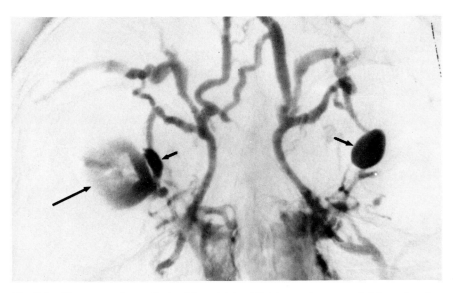

Fig. 2-1. Venogram of a patient with a right orbital hemorrhage reveals bilateral varices (short arrows). The hemorrhage originates from the ruptured right varix and is defined by the contrast material extravasating into the muscle cone (long arrow). From Krohel GB, Wright JE: Orbital hemorrhage. Am J Ophthalmol 80:254, 1979.

The traumatic hemorrhages are usually associated with orbital fractures. Visual loss may be secondary to the compressive effects of the hemorrhage or due to an associated optic canal fracture. The possibility of postoperative orbital hemorrhage with visual loss must always be considered in the patient with severe postoperative pain following eyelid or orbital surgery.

Orbital Cellulitis

Orbital cellulitis most commonly arises from organisms that gain access to the orbit from the contiguous paranasal sinuses, lids, or mouth. Other etiologies include trauma, insect bites, and hematogenous spread of infection. The usual pathogens cultured are *Staphylococcus aureus, Streptococcus pyogenes, Escherichia coli, Streptococcus pneumoniae,* and *Hemophilus influenzae* type B.

Inflammation anterior to the orbital septum (preseptal, anterior orbital cellulitis) presents with lid swelling and erythema. Inflammation posterior to the septum (posterior orbital cellulitis) is signaled by the additional findings of chemosis, proptosis, motility disturbance, or visual loss. The pain usually develops fairly rapidly and subsides several days after institution of appropriate antibiotic therapy. Progression of symptoms may indicate formation of an orbital abscess. Cellulitis can occur at any age but is more common in children.

Inflammatory Orbital Pseudotumor

This label should not be attached to inflammatory orbital diseases of known etiology, such as vasculitis with polyarteritis nodosa or foreign body reaction; when possible, these disease processes should be categorized according to their

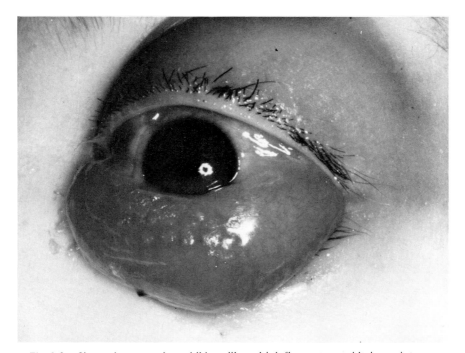

Fig. 2-2. Chemosis, proptosis, and lid swelling with inflammatory orbital pseudotumor.

appropriate etiologies. The nonspecific term "inflammatory orbital pseudo-tumor" should be used only in those patients with orbital inflammatory syndrome in whom an etiologic diagnosis is not possible. The etiology of most inflammatory orbital processes remains obscure but probably involves an immunologic abnormality. Pain, proptosis, motility disturbance, lid swelling, and injection are the hallmarks of this condition (Fig. 2-2). Patients with periosteal involvement may have severe pain, whereas anterior orbital lesions may produce only slight discomfort. Patients with recurring orbital pseudotumor will often be pain-free with exacerbations of pain noted during bouts of upper respiratory infection. Patients with an inflammatory process involving the orbital apex or cavernous sinus (Tolosa-Hunt syndrome) have severe pain. Inflammatory orbital pseudotumor in any location is usually sensitive to treatment with corticosteroids.

Posterior Scleritis

The pain associated with posterior scleritis is often located deep in the orbit, with radiation to the temple. There is often a mild amount of proptosis and injection. An anterior chamber reaction may be present. The presence of localized choroidal effusions may help differentiate posterior scleritis from orbital pseudotumor. Indirect funduscopy through a dilated pupil is, therefore, essential in the workup of all orbital patients. Posterior scleritis is often associated with systemic diseases such as rheumatoid arthritis, polyarteritis nodosa, herpes zoster, syphilis, or tuberculosis.

Malignant Lacrimal Gland Tumors

These tumors will frequently cause a deep, gnawing, orbital pain at some time during their course. The pain may be episodic, and some of these patients may be treated for headaches before the real etiology is discovered. Adenoid cystic carcinomas can produce pain before a large mass is appreciated, due to submucosal growth with perineural invasion. An associated loss of sensation in the distribution of the lacrimal nerve can occur. There is often a palpable mass in the superior temporal quadrant of the orbit. The evolution of symptoms becomes apparent over several months. Pain often signals a bad prognosis indicating periosteal or bony involvement. The dismal prognosis of these tumors demands an aggressive approach to early diagnosis and treatment.

LESIONS LESS FREQUENTLY PAINFUL

These types of lesions cause pain in less than 75 percent of cases.

Orbital Abscess

Abscess formation usually results from spread of a subperiosteal abscess, localization of an orbital cellulitis, or contamination by a foreign body. Partially treated cases of orbital abscess may present as a mass lesion. In these cases the local inflammatory signs and leukocytosis are masked by the antibiotics. Relief of pain follows surgical incision and drainage.

Metastatic Disease in Adults

Pain occurs in approximately 30 percent of patients with metastatic orbital tumors. The onset is often acute. Other signs such as ptosis, visual loss, lid swelling, proptosis, motility disturbance, and diplopia depend on the site of metastases. The most common sites of primary tumors in adults include the breast, lung, and kidney. These tumors may metastasize many years after discovery of the primary tumor. Breast carcinomas in particular may present ten to twenty years after their initial resection.

Metastatic Disease in Children

This category includes neuroblastoma, granulocytic sarcoma (chloroma) with leukemia, Ewing's sarcoma, and, rarely, Wilm's tumor. Neuroblastoma usually occurs before age 4. The median age for granulocytic sarcoma is 7, and Ewing's sarcoma usually occurs between ages 10 and 25. All of these tumors can invade bony structures. In addition, neuroblastoma, Ewing's sarcoma, and granulocytic sarcoma can necrose blood vessels, producing an orbital hemorrhage with lid ecchymosis.

Phycomycosis

Orbital fungal infections produce acute proptosis, visual loss, and ophthalmoplegia. Diabetic patients in metabolic acidosis and immunosuppressed patients are especially vulnerable. Orbital pain is present in approximately 20 percent of these cases. Other clinical signs include central retinal artery occlusion, chemosis, periorbital discoloration, altered mental status, palatal eschar, and involvement of cranial nerves II through VII.

The responsible fungus (usually *Mucor* or *Rhizopus*) is initially found in the palate or paranasal sinuses and rapidly spreads to the orbit. The fungus invades arteries, causing thrombosis and subsequent tissue infarction.

Osteogenic Sarcoma

These tumors can arise in the skull or maxilla, with secondary invasion of the orbit. There is probably a genetic predisposition towards development of osteogenic sarcoma in patients with bilateral retinoblastoma. Previous radiotherapy may be a contributing etiologic factor. Local swelling and numbness are the initial complaints. Pain usually occurs late in the disease. Males in the third decade have the highest incidence.

Arteriovenous Malformations

Carotid-cavernous sinus fistulas are the type of arteriovenous malformation (AVM) most commonly encountered. Orbital pain occurs in about 20 percent of these patients. Pain in carotid-cavernous sinus fistulas is often secondary to ocular ischemia or glaucoma. The fistulas usually result from trauma, but spontaneous fistulas also occur. Other findings include subjective bruit, proptosis, motility disturbance, episcleral injection, and visual loss. Orbital AVMs are less common. Fistulas can also occur between dural vessels and meningeal arterial branches. These usually have an insidious, uncomplicated course and frequently undergo spontaneous resolution.

LESIONS INFREQUENTLY PAINFUL

These lesions are associated with pain in less than 10 percent of cases.

Sinus Mucocele

The most common location for sinus mucoceles is the frontal and ethmoidal sinuses, although sphenoidal and maxillary sinus mucoceles do occur. With frontal sinus involvement the patients are usually pain-free unless there is an associated infection. Patients may complain of intermittent burning, tearing, and injection. Physical findings, which are based on the location of the mucocele, include muscle imbalance, proptosis, globe displacement, and optic atrophy. Pain or headache is more common with sphenoidal and ethmoidal mucoceles. Pain may be episodic, and migraine attacks may be simulated by sphenoidal mucoceles. In addition, sphenoidal mucoceles may produce third nerve palsy and optic atrophy. The underlying mechanism of mucocele formation is sinus blockage secondary to obstruction of the ostium. This can occur secondary to chronic sinusitis, congenital malformations of the sinus, fractures, and tumors.

Thyroid Ophthalmopathy

Thyroid ophthalmopathy is a common cause of abnormal orbital findings, and most patients do not have severe pain. Patients with severe corneal exposure will complain of burning, tearing, and the sensation of a foreign body in the eye. Erosion of the cornea secondary to exposure may produce severe discomfort (Fig. 2-3). In addition, patients may complain of a pulling or tightness of the orbit on extreme abduction or elevation, secondary to rectus muscle restriction. Lid swelling or fullness and conjunctival swelling (chemosis) are frequent complaints. They are often worse in the morning and may be accompanied by transient diplopia, which improves after an hour or so. Constant orbital pain in the primary position in the absence of corneal exposure should make one suspicious of another disease process. The etiology of thyroid ophthalmopathy remains obscure. Thyroid patients can be chemically euthyroid, hyperthyroid, or hypothyroid. Most patients eventually develop clinical or chemical evidence of thyroid disease.

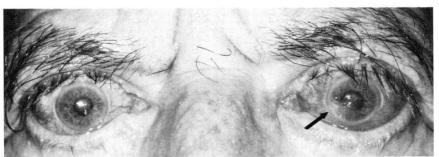

Fig. 2-3. Lid retraction and proptosis in a patient with thyroid ophthalmopathy. Severe left-sided ocular pain was secondary to erosion of the cornea inferiorly (arrow).

Cavernous Hemangioma

These vascular tumors occur in the second to the fifth decade of life. They undergo slow progressive enlargement over years, with motility disturbance, proptosis, indentation of the globe, and eventual visual loss. They often arise intraconally between the optic nerve and lateral rectus muscle. Pain is rare unless corneal exposure is present.

Capillary Hemangioma

Unlike cavernous hemangiomas, these tumors occur primarily in the first year of life and tend to involute after an initial period of enlargement. They are usually present in the lids, anterior orbit, and outside the muscle cone. Histopathologically, capillary hemangiomas contain pericytes, macrophages, and endothelial cells and have small vascular lumens. This contrasts with the large lumens, flattened endothelial cells, and smooth muscle cells seen microscopically in a cavernous hemangioma. Pain is uncommon but may occur when a lid lesion undergoes spontaneous ulceration or necrosis.

Varix

Patients with orbital varices generally do not have pain. Patients may experience a pressure sensation around the eye when the orbital veins become engorged such as with a Valsalva maneuver. Severe orbital pain can occur with a secondary orbital hemorrhage, but this is less common.

Benign Mixed Lacrimal Gland Tumor
(Pleomorphic Adenoma)

Pain occurs in approximately 5 percent of patients with pleomorphic adenoma. Patients with malignant lacrimal gland tumors, in contrast, frequently complain of pain at some time in the course of the disease. Age of onset varies from the late twenties to the fifties. The clinical course is characteristically prolonged (longer than 12 months).

Fibrous Histiocytoma

In recent years, this locally invasive, spindle cell tumor of mesenchymal origin has been diagnosed with increased frequency. This tumor may occur at any age. Proptosis and motility disturbances are frequently seen. Pain is rare even with tumor recurrence. Central nervous system invasion can occur by relentless local spread and may produce discomfort late in the course of the disease. Metastases are rare.

Dermoid Cyst

These lesions represent tumefactions of tissue of ectodermal origin, and they may arise from conjunctival or cutaneous sites. Patients with dermoid cysts may complain of mild intermittent burning or irritation. Rupture of a dermoid cyst can incite a severe granulomatous inflammatory response clinically similar to inflammatory orbital pseudotumor. In general, however, patients with dermoids do not complain of pain, although the lesions are usually present for many years. They are more common in childhood but will occasionally be noted for the first time in adulthood. Review of old photographs in these adults will often reveal orbital asymmetry indicative of a long-standing process.

Rhabdomyosarcoma

This rapidly growing neoplasm produces pain in approximately 10 percent of patients. The mass can assume huge proportions if neglected, and pain is more common in such cases. In addition to proptosis, patients may present with a lid or subconjunctival mass. Most cases present in the first decade of life. Nosebleeds and visual loss are less common modes of presentation.

Lymphoma

Orbital lymphoma, histiocytic lymphoma, and Hodgkins-type lymphoma are generally painless masses. In addition, pain is uncommon with orbital involvement secondary to sinus histiocytosis and Burkitt's lymphoma.

Osseous Tumors

These lesions are generally painless, with the exception of osteogenic sarcoma. Included in this category are fibrous dysplasia, ossifying fibroma, osteoblastoma, aneurysmal bone cyst, diaphyseal dysplasia (Englemann's disease), and other craniofacial dysostoses. Osteomas cause pain in roughly 5 percent of patients. They usually arise in middle age and can involve frontal, sphenoid, ethmoid, or maxillary sinuses. Exophthalmos, facial asymmetry, nasal obstruction, and optic atrophy can occur. Occasionally, osteomas may be inherited in a dominant fashion with associated epidermoid cysts, fibromas, and polyps of the colon (Gardner's syndrome).

Arachnoidal Cysts

These uncommon lesions are painless when confined to the orbital portion of the optic nerve. Pain or chronic headache is often reported with intracranial cysts extending into the orbit.

Neurogenic Tumors

Included in this category are neurofibromas, neurilemomas, gliomas, and meningiomas. Although tumors are generally painless, pain may occur in the following cases: Neurilemomas can produce pain occasionally by compression of an orbital nerve. Malignant transformation of a neurilemoma or neurofibroma (rare) can result in pain. In addition, isolated neurofibromas arising from the nasociliary nerves can cause chronic pain. Sphenoid meningiomas can invade the orbit and produce pain in advanced cases or where there has been sarcomatous change. Primary intraorbital meningiomas do not usually cause pain, and the presence of pain often signals invasion of the optic canal or cranium.

Basal Cell Carcinoma

These lesions are usually painless, even with massive destruction of the globe and orbit. This is probably due to concomitant destruction of sensory nerves (Fig. 2-4).

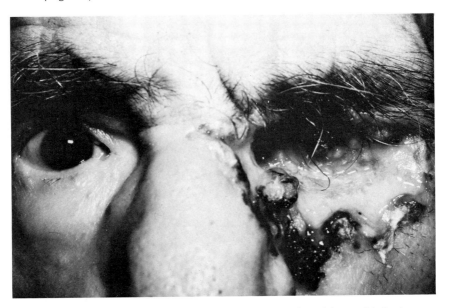

Fig. 2-4.   A basal cell carcinoma producing tissue destruction without orbital pain.

3
The Six P's of Orbital
Clinical Evaluation: Progression

The second "P" of orbital disease is Progression, which should remind us to question the patient carefully about the onset, duration, and course of his or her symptoms.

Rapidity of onset is an important marker of orbital disease. Inspection of old photographs and historical data from family members or friends can be extremely useful when the patient is not a reliable historian. With such a patient, the clinician may gain more information on duration of symptoms by noting whether or not diplopia is present in the primary position. A patient with a displaced globe secondary to a slowly growing tumor (years) will usually not report diplopia in primary position. In contrast, the patient in whom globe displacement occurs over weeks to months will almost always report diplopia in the primary position. The exception occurs in children, where visual suppression will usually "protect" the patient from diplopia with both acute and chronic globe displacement.

RAPID ONSET (DAYS TO WEEKS)

In general, acute lesions are often associated with tenderness on palpation as well as diplopia. Rapidly evolving lesions, such as orbital hemorrhage, may also produce nausea and vomiting secondary to a vasovagal reaction.

Orbital Cellulitis

With orbital cellulitis, rapid onset over several days is the rule, except in immunosuppressed patients who may have an insidious course mimicking an orbital neoplasm.

Orbital Pseudotumor

Approximately 75 percent of patients will note onset of symptoms over a one-week period.

Orbital Thrombophlebitis

Onset of symptoms usually occurs within 24 hours. Patients are often quite ill. The symptom complex often simulates cellulitis or acute inflammatory orbital pseudotumor. Most cases are secondary to orbital infection or thrombosis of arteriovenous fistulas.

Orbital Hemorrhage

Both traumatic and spontaneous hemorrhages usually occur over several hours. A small hemorrhage will occasionally be lined by endothelial cells of venous or lymphatic origin and will undergo progressive enlargement. Thus, a slowly progressive mass lesion is simulated. These "blood cysts" occur more commonly in children.

Rhabdomyosarcoma

Symptoms usually develop over a one- to two-week period. Parents of affected children may report a history of seemingly trivial trauma and will blame the ecchymosis or proptosis on this. The rapid evolution of symptoms should deter the physician from accepting this "false-positive" history.

Metastatic Disease in Children

Both neuroblastoma and granulocytic sarcoma (leukemia) are noted for their rapid onset of proptosis. These rapidly growing tumors can infiltrate blood vessels, producing infarction and necrosis.

GRADUAL ONSET (MONTHS TO YEARS)

Dermoid Cyst

These cystic tumors are usually first noted in childhood. Some escape early detection and are not picked up until adulthood. They are generally slow-growing tumors and may not change clinically over several years.

Benign Mixed Lacrimal Gland Tumor

Patients usually provide a history dating the disease process to more than one year. Inspection of old photographs can be helpful. The surgical approach to lacrimal gland fossa tumors (biopsy versus excision) often rests upon the history alone, as the physical examination of benign and malignant tumors often results in similar findings.

Neurogenic Tumor

Glioma, meningioma, neurilemomma, and neurofibroma are included in this category. These tumors usually exhibit slow growth over many months unless there has been sarcomatous degeneration, which is rare.

Cavernous Hemangioma

These are usually slow-growing tumors, with symptoms developing over several years. Occasionally growth is more rapid, especially during pregnancy. Hemangiomas may remain relatively dormant for years in older patients. They typically produce proptosis first and visual loss later, in contrast to optic nerve sheath meningiomas, in which visual loss may be the presenting complaint.

Fibrous Histiocytoma

These are generally slow-growing tumors that tend to recur if not completely excised. A recurrence can occur many years after initial surgery. Despite slow growth, diplopia can occur secondary to infiltration of the extraocular muscles.

Osseous Tumors

Osteoma and fibrous dysplasia typically produce facial asymmetry and proptosis over months to years.

VARIABLE ONSET

Lymphoma

Well-differentiated lymphomas usually present over several months with proptosis and anteriorly palpable masses. Poorly differentiated lymphocytic tumors and some histiocytic lymphomas may have a more fulminant course.

Sinus Mucocele

Mucoceles usually have an insidious onset. Some become infected (pyoceles), in which case the onset is acute and associated with proptosis, displacement of the globe, and pain.

Arteriovenous (AV) Malformation

Large AV malformations, such as carotid cavernous fistulas, usually present over several weeks. Secondary traumatic fistulas may present days to months after the accident. Smaller fistulas may have a more chronic course with evolution of symptoms over several months. Thrombosis of the orbital veins can produce a more abrupt and dramatic increase in proptosis.

Metastatic Disease in Adults

The two most common sites of origin are the breasts in women and the lungs in men. Patients frequently present with acute or subacute lid swelling, proptosis, diplopia, and pain. Some patients exhibit a less fulminant course with diplopia or minimal proptosis appearing over many months.

Thyroid Ophthalmopathy

Symptoms can usually be elicited over a several-month period. Minor symptoms such as lid swelling, lid erythema, or tearing are often overlooked by the patient and physician. Some patients complain of vague discomfort on upgaze, increased prominence of the eyes, and diplopia (especially in the morning hours and associated with close work). It is not rare, however, for a patient to suddenly experience constant diplopia. A careful history will reveal that there has been intermittent diplopia or blurring over the preceding weeks. In addition, some patients have acute episodes of visual loss and discomfort secondary to corneal breakdown. The key to correct diagnosis is the vague but persistent symptoms mentioned above, which are usually present for weeks or months.

Varix

Most patients have a history of recurrent short-lived proptosis or lid swelling over months to years. This is often brought on by Valsalva's maneuver (such as crying or straining). A patient with AV malformation may develop an orbital hemorrhage, in which case there is sudden pain and nausea in addition to proptosis.

Malignant Lacrimal Gland Tumor

A patient with such a tumor usually has symptoms of less than one year's duration. This factor, along with the frequent occurrence of pain, helps clinically separate malignant tumors from the benign mixed type.

Capillary Hemangioma

These tumors are often present at birth and undergo enlargement in the first year of life. Occasionally, more rapid growth over several weeks will mimic the presentation of rhabdomyosarcoma.

4

The Six P's of Orbital
Clinical Evaluation: Proptosis

Proptosis, a forward protrusion or bulging of the globe, is related to the physical examination rather than to the history, and is the hallmark of orbital disease.

Questions are commonly raised about the significance of exophthalmometer readings. Values ranging from 20 to 24 mm have been considered abnormal by various authors. This wide range clearly indicates that no clear definition of proptosis can be based on measurements alone. Measurements merely contribute to the evaluation of the problem and provide an objective method of following a patient. Similarly, a difference of greater than 2 mm between eyes is considered abnormal and an indication for an orbital workup. Asymmetry of readings, however, does not necessarily imply that true proptosis is present.

The most valuable instrument in the diagnosis of subtle proptosis is not the exophthalmometer but rather an old photograph (e.g., a driver's license with an attached photo). Review of old serial photographs may allow recognition of subtle changes in appearance that may not be apparent to the patient. Allowance also must be made for racial differences (many black people have very prominent eyes), familial variations, and normal hemifacial asymmetry.

PSEUDOPROPTOSIS

Certain orbital and ocular asymmetries may lead to a false impression of proptosis or "pseudoproptosis." Pseudoproptosis must first be ruled out in every patient. Causes of pseudoproptosis include asymmetry of bony orbits, enlarged globe, asymmetry of the lid fissures, relaxation of rectus muscles, and contralateral enophthalmos.

Asymmetry of Bony Orbits

Such asymmetry may be due to trauma, irradiation, or surgery, or it may be congenital or hereditary. Every patient should be questioned carefully about previous trauma. It is also important to note prior activities and occupations. Some patients (football players, boxers, etc.) are not aware that they have sustained facial fractures in the past.

Patients who have been treated with local irradiation or who have had orbital bone surgery before age 8 may have retarded growth of the orbital bones with resultant relative enophthalmos. Similarly, a child who has undergone enucleation may have a small socket, even if orbital expansion procedures are carried out postoperatively.

Enlarged Globe

This condition may be caused by myopia or buphthalmos. Ultrasonography with A-scan technique is the most useful tool to demonstrate an abnormal elongation of the globe, especially in patients with media opacities.

Asymmetry of the Lid Fissures

This condition may be due to lid retraction, ptosis, or seventh cranial nerve paralysis. Lid retraction, such as that seen in thyroid disease, can simulate the appearance of proptosis or accentuate a preexisting proptosis. Patients with ptosis can appear enophthalmic on the affected side (Fig. 4-1). Patients with unilateral ptosis involving the dominant eye often have secondary overaction of the opposite levator muscle due to Hering's law of innervation. This can produce lid retraction on the opposite side, with resultant pseudoproptosis. Mechanical elevation of the ptotic lid or patching of that side may eliminate the added innervation and relieve the lid retraction. Seventh nerve paralysis may cause widening of the palpebral fissure with abnormal exposure of sclera, which simulates proptosis.

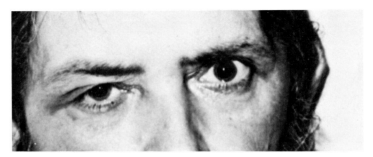

Fig. 4-1. Metastatic lung carcinoma to the right orbit, producing blepharoptosis and apparent enophthalmos. The patient was initially referred for proptosis of the left eye.

Relaxation of Rectus Muscles

One to two millimeters of proptosis can result from third cranial nerve palsy or surgical muscle recessions.

Contralateral Enophthalmos

Bone defects in neurofibromatosis can lead to enophthalmos when there are no concomitant orbital tumors. A condition such as phthisis bulbi or microphthalmos may lead one to suspect proptosis of the fellow eye. Metastatic scirrhous breast carcinoma may incite a fibrotic reaction, with subsequent enophthalmos rather than exophthalmos of the affected orbit (Fig. 4-2).

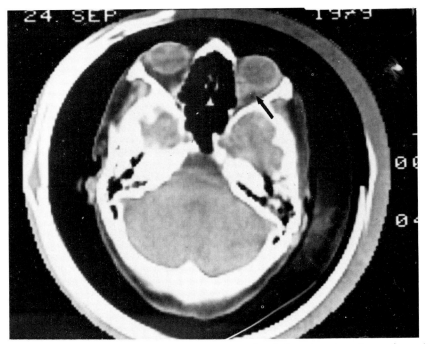

Fig. 4-2. Left globe retraction secondary to metastatic scirrhous breast carcinoma (arrow). The patient was initially referred for proptosis of the right eye.

BILATERAL PROPTOSIS

This diagnostic category may suggest any one of a variety of conditions.

Thyroid Ophthalmopathy

This is certainly the most frequent cause of both unilateral and bilateral proptosis in adults.

Carotid-Cavernous Sinus Fistulas

These patients may develop bilateral proptosis with bruits, although the involvement is often asymmetric (Fig. 4-3).

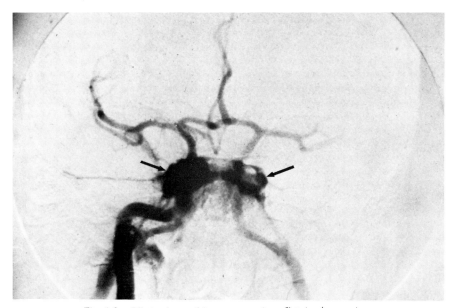

Fig. 4-3.   Bilateral carotid cavernous sinus fistulas (arrows).

Cavernous Sinus Thrombosis

The septic form is usually bilateral, fulminant, and often fatal. The aseptic type may occur secondary to arteriovenous fistulas and is often bilateral.

Vasculitis

Wegener's granulomatosis is probably the most common disease in this group. Bilateral proptosis, which may be responsive to steroids, radiotherapy, or cytotoxic agents, is the rule (Fig. 4-4).

Inflammatory Pseudotumor

Many patients with this condition belong in the vasculitis category. Some patients with predominantly lymphocytic pseudotumors eventually develop systemic manifestations of lymphoma. There is a small group of patients, how-

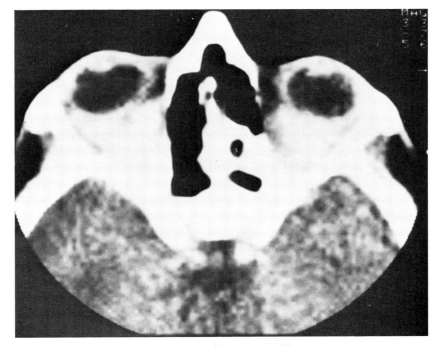

Fig. 4-4. Diffuse bilateral orbital infiltration with Wegener's granulomatosis.

ever, who manifest bilateral involvement with idiopathic inflammatory pseudo-tumor. This is more common in the second and third decades of life. There is usually some separation in time between involvement of each orbit.

Lymphoma

Bilateral involvement may occur.

Leukemia

Bilateral proptosis, often acute, can occur in children.

Neuroblastoma

Bilateral involvement occurs in over 50% of cases.

Craniofacial Dysostosis

Crouzon's disease and other congenital orbital malformations can result in bilateral proptosis with associated optic atrophy, strabismus, and nystagmus.

RECURRENT PROPTOSIS

Venous Anomalies

Orbital varices are the most common cause of intermittent proptosis. Most varices are primary and first appear in childhood. Some occur secondary to intracranial or intraorbital arteriovenous malformations. The proptosis can often be reproduced by having the patient perform a Valsalva's maneuver. Some patients, especially those with long-standing varices, show no evidence of increased proptosis with Valsalva's maneuver. The varix is presumably closed off from the venous circulation by a previous thrombosis, hemorrhage, or inflammatory process.

Table 4-1
Differentiation of Varices, Lymphangiomas, and Capillary Hemangiomas

Clinicopathologic Findings	Varices	Lymphangiomas	Capillary Hemangiomas
Intermittent proptosis	Yes	Yes	Uncommon
Increased proptosis with Valsalva's maneuver	Yes	Yes	Yes
Vascular anomalies of palate and head	Yes	Yes	Yes
Visible cutaneous vascular anomalies	Yes	Yes	Yes
Spontaneous orbital hemorrhage	Yes	Yes	No
Exacerbation with URI	No	Yes	No
Response to radiotherapy	No	No	Yes
Response to corticosteroids	No	No	Yes
Venography	Positive	Negative	Negative
Enlarged orbit on skull x-ray	Yes	Yes	Yes
Phleboliths on skull x-ray	Yes	No	Uncommon
Endothelial lined spaces pathologically	Yes	Yes	Yes
Smooth muscle cells on electron microscopy	Yes	No	No
Can occur secondary to AV fistulas	Yes	No	Uncommon
Can evolve into chronic blood cysts	Yes	Yes	No
During ultrasound, size increases with compression of the jugular vein	Occasionally	No	No
Association with Klippel Trenaunay Weber syndrome	Yes	No	No
Can produce amblyopia	Yes	Yes	Yes

Lymphangioma

A debate exists on whether patients with recurrent proptosis, hemorrhage, and visible vascular lesions have orbital varices or lymphangioma. The debate centers on physical examination findings, radiologic (venography) observations, and histopathologic aspects including electron microscopy. Fortunately for the practitioner, the debate is largely academic, as the treatment and course of such patients is not generally changed by the label one attaches to their disease. Table 4-1 compares the features of varices, lymphangiomas and capillary hemangiomas. Capillary hemangiomas are included in the table because of their frequent confusion with other vascular lesions. The distinction is crucial, as capillary hemangiomas, in contrast to varices or lymphangiomas, may be amenable to treatment with corticosteroids and irradiation.

Inflammatory Pseudotumor

Exacerbations of inflammatory pseudotumor may occur. Some patients may experience intervals of over 10 years between attacks.

Sinus Mucoceles

Mucoceles may become secondarily infected (pyoceles), with increased proptosis, erythema, and pain. In addition, the patient may experience intermittent irritation and discomfort when the ostium becomes completely occluded and the sinus is distended. Partial opening of the ostium or bony expansion may then afford temporary pain relief.

Dermoid Cysts

Incompletely excised dermoids can continue to leak material, which may set up a granulomatous inflammatory response. In such a case, the recurrent episodes may be quite fulminant, with a dramatic increase in proptosis, pain, and injection.

DIRECTION OF GLOBE DISPLACEMENT

As with many diagnostic signs in orbital disease, globe displacement can help narrow the diagnostic possibilities. Masses within the muscle cone produce axial proptosis, whereas superior nasal masses push the eye downward and laterally. Inferior orbital masses usually push the globe upward, with limitation of supraduction or infraduction. In such cases, poor downgaze can result from mass effect, whereas decreased upward gaze may result from tethering of the inferior rectus muscle by the mass.

AXIAL DISPLACEMENT

Cavernous Hemangioma

This is the most common primary orbital tumor encountered in adults, and it usually arises laterally in the muscle cone (Fig. 4-5).

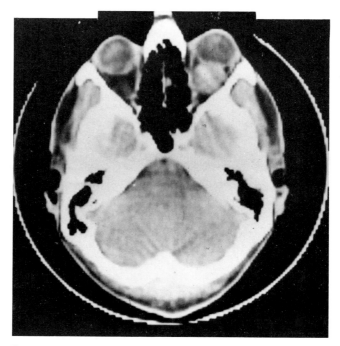

Fig. 4-5. Cavernous hemangioma of the left orbit. This encapsulated tumor arises within the muscle cone and produces axial proptosis. There is usually a clear space between the posterior wall of the tumor and the bony orbital apex.

Neurilemoma

The majority of neurilemomas occur in the muscle cone, producing axial displacement. The second most common location is the superior orbit, in which case the globe is displaced downward.

Optic Nerve Glioma

Axial displacement is the rule initially. Later in the course of the disease, the eye is usually displaced downwards.

Meningioma

Optic nerve sheath meningiomas produce delayed and subtle axial proptosis, especially when located posteriorly. Visual loss usually occurs early in the course of the disease. Sphenoid wing meningiomas, in contrast, can produce massive proptosis with downward globe displacement.

Arteriovenous Malformations

Axial proptosis with significant chemosis and "red eye" are the usual presenting signs (Fig. 4-6). This usually becomes a bilateral disease because of the rich anastomosis between venous channels.

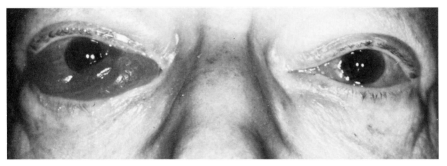

Fig. 4-6. Bilateral chemosis, injection and axial proptosis with an arteriovenous malformation. The patient was initially thought to have thyroid ophthalmopathy.

Metastatic Tumors

The proptosis is frequently axial, even though half of these tumors metastasize to the superior orbit. Downward displacement is the second most common presentation. Ocular rotations are often limited.

SUPERIOR DISPLACEMENT

Maxillary Sinus Tumors

These tumors may produce upward globe displacement late in the course of the disease, after orbital extension has occurred. Pain and inferior chemosis may be present.

Fibromatosis

These firm, painless tumors usually occur in childhood.

DOWNWARD DISPLACEMENT

Thyroid Ophthalmopathy

This is the most common cause of downward displacement of the globe. The etiology is fibrosis and restriction of the inferior rectus muscle. The next most common presentation is medial globe retraction, which produces an esotropia. Occasionally, superior displacement secondary to predominant involvement of the superior rectus muscle will be seen.

Dermoid Cysts

These tumors usually present superiorly in the orbit, either laterally or medially (Fig. 4-7). There is often no globe displacement in children. Large cysts can insidiously push the globe inferiorly in adults.

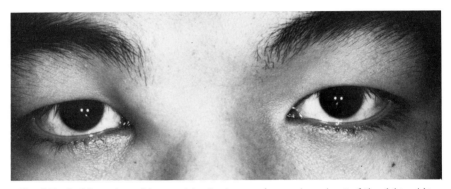

Fig. 4-7. Insidious dermoid cyst arising in the superior nasal quadrant of the right orbit.

Capillary Hemangioma

In distinction to cavernous hemangiomas of adults with purely axial proptosis, these tumors often involve the upper orbit, with resultant downward and axial displacement. Involvement of the upper lid can produce irregular astigmatism with resultant anisometropic amblyopia.

Lacrimal Gland Tumors

Displacement is usually downward and inward. Other tumors involving the lacrimal gland fossa include metastatic lesions, lymphoma, inflammatory pseudotumor, and dermoids.

Neuroblastoma

These tumors have a tendency to metastasize to the zygomatic bone, producing medial displacement with either an axial or downward component.

Frontal Sinus Mucocele

These patients often have downward and lateral displacement of the globe, as most mucoceles involve the frontal or ethmoidal sinus (Fig. 4-8).

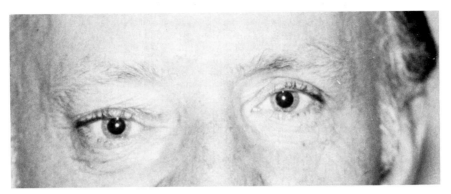

Fig. 4-8. Downward and lateral displacement of the right globe with a frontal sinus mucocele.

Orbital Abscess

Displacement naturally depends on location of the abscess. Orbital abscesses frequently occur secondary to frontal or ethmoidal sinus disease, producing downward and lateral globe displacement.

Neurofibromas

These can be divided into two types: (1) the plexiform, diffuse type, and (2) the solitary, circumscribed type. The solitary neurofibromas occur either anteriorly and medially, or superotemporally in the muscle cone. An isolated neurofibroma will often arise from branches of the nasociliary nerve as it leaves the superior orbital fissure, with axial and downward displacement.

Plexiform neurofibromas are associated with neurofibromatosis, and they diffusely infiltrate the orbit and lids. The globe is often displaced downward and laterally. Significant facial deformities may occur.

Osteoma

These tumors are most commonly encountered in the frontal or ethmoidal sinus. Displacement of the globe is often downward and lateral, and it usually becomes apparent over a rather long period of time. Sphenoid sinus osteomas produce orbital symptoms late in their course. Maxillary tumors may displace the globe upward. Most osteomas, however, are asymptomatic and do not produce globe displacement.

Frontal Sinus Tumors

These are uncommon. They may mimic sinus mucoceles in presentation.

Fibrous Dysplasia

Displacement is inferior in approximately 40 percent of cases, due to frequent involvement of the frontal bone. Sphenoid, ethmoid, zygomatic, and maxillary involvement does occur and, of course, changes the pattern of displacement. Concomitant facial deformity usually develops over many years.

Rhabdomyosarcoma

Most cases initially have axial proptosis, although approximately 20 percent exhibit downward and outward displacement (Fig. 4-9). Downward globe displacement is usually evident in more advanced cases.

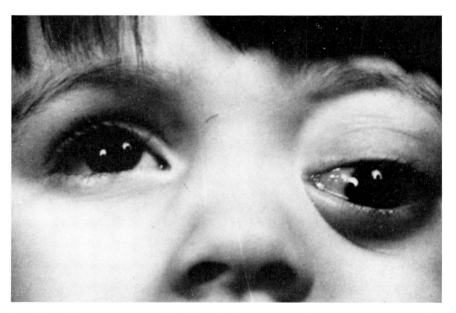

Fig. 4-9. Rhabdomyosarcoma of the left orbit, displacing the globe downward and laterally.

Lymphoma and Pseudotumor

Both lymphoma and pseudotumor may present anywhere in the orbit. Although the superior quadrant is the most common location (producing downward globe displacement), a significant number of these masses do occur in the inferior orbital space, producing upward globe displacement, and in the muscle cone, producing axial proptosis. Therefore, when confronted with upward globe displacement, the most likely diagnosis is lymphoma or pseudotumor. These are both common diseases, and although the inferior orbit is not the most frequent site of occurrence, they still outnumber the other lesions that produce superior globe displacement.

5
The Six P's of Orbital
Clinical Evaluation: Palpation

Palpation, although restricted in the amount of information it can provide, is a useful and necessary part of the physical examination of the orbit. Palpation of the orbit is most effective when the patient keeps the eyelids open and maintains gaze in primary position. One must resist the temptation of having the patient look down when palpating the superior orbit. This will often tighten the orbital septum, precluding deep palpation by the examiner. One is generally unable to palpate masses posterior to the equator of the globe. Thus, anterior orbital masses (anterior to the equator of the globe) are fully or partially palpable, whereas the more posterior masses are characterized by proptosis and increased resistance to retropulsion of the globe.

The ideal time to palpate the orbit is after induction of general anesthesia. With orbital relaxation the examiner can often discern deep masses, especially in children.

Resistance to retropulsion of the globe has often been described as a hallmark of thyroid ophthalmopathy. However, other infiltrative inflammatory processes as well as solid and cystic tumors can cause significant resistance to ocular retropulsion.

The lacrimal gland may be pushed forward in many cases of proptosis. One must be alert to this possibility when palpating around the lacrimal fossa and when a biopsy is taken from this area. Biopsy by the unwary surgeon may result in excision of normal lacrimal gland instead of the tumor, which lurks deeper in the orbit. Similarly, orbital fat may also be displaced anteriorly by a posterior mass.

Palpation can be helpful in planning the surgical approach. Finally, the presence or absence of tenderness, induration or fluctuance may be confirmed by orbital palpation.

39

SUPERIOR NASAL QUADRANT

Sinus Mucocele

One often encounters a smooth-walled fluctuant mass, which can be described as "boggy" to palpation. Crepitance is occasionally appreciated. Tenderness is present when there is an inflammatory component. Marked tenderness on palpation is encountered when the sac is infected (pyocele).

Dermoid Cysts

These cysts are usually smooth and firm. In children they are located anteriorly, are oval in configuration, and are freely movable. In adults, only the anterior portion may be palpated. Tenderness is present in some cases, especially along eroded bone. Incompletely excised or ruptured dermoids can cause a marked inflammatory reaction and tenderness on palpation.

Encephalocele

This diagnosis should be entertained when any midline mass is encountered in infancy. The mass is often fluctuant to palpation and may transilluminate. Encephalocele can be associated with optic nerve abnormalities such as optic nerve dysplasia or coloboma.

Fibrous Histiocytoma

These tumors may initially be cystic to palpation when anterior in location. Incomplete excision is common as tissue borders are ill-defined. On recurrence,

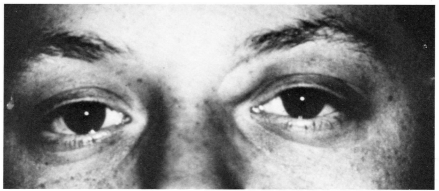

Fig. 5-1. Recurrent fibrous histiocytoma in the upper nasal quadrant of the left orbit. A surgical scar from a previous surgical excision is evident. (From Krohel GB, Gregor Z: Fibrous histiocytoma. Journal of Pediatric Ophthalmology and Strabismus 17:37,1980.)

the characteristics on palpation are markedly different. The recurrent fibrous histiocytomas are firm and immovable and often attach to underlying periosteum. They are often located in the superior and medial portions of the orbit (Fig. 5-1).

Solitary Neurofibroma

These tumors either appear in the superior temporal orbit, where they are not palpable or in the anterior medial aspect of the orbit. When located anteriorly they feel firm but not rock-hard.

Plexiform Neurofibroma

This tumor is known as a "bag of worms," and no other description can be more accurately applied. The tumor is usually diffuse and often involves the levator aponeurosis. It can be palpated deep into the orbit, as the septum is often replaced or attenuated by the mass.

Metastatic Tumors in Adults

These tumors occur in the superior quadrants in approximately 60 percent of cases. They can often be palpated in the superior nasal quadrant, where they may be fixed to bone and/or trochlea. They are often rock-hard and are tender when there has been periosteal or bone invasion.

Osteoma

Osteomas are often too deep to palpate. Large anterior tumors (frontal or ethmoidal) are rock-hard to palpation.

Capillary Hemangioma

Approximately one third of capillary hemangiomas involve the upper nasal quadrant. The lid and anterior orbital portions are palpable and compressible.

Lymphoma

Lymphomas will often be palpable along the entire superior aspect of the orbit. They are firm to palpation and are *not* fixed to bone.

SUPERIOR TEMPORAL QUADRANT

Inflammatory Pseudotumor

Inflammatory pseudotumor is often indistinguishable from lymphoma by palpation; however, distinction may be made in that pseudotumors are often tender to palpation and associated with inflammatory signs.

Epithelial Lacrimal Gland Tumors

These tumors are firm to palpation and are often fixed to the bony margins. They may be distinguished from pseudotumor and lymphomas by the presence of characteristic changes on plain skull x-rays. (See Chapter 6.) Lymphomas, dermoid cysts, metastases and inflammatory pseudotumors can occur in the superior nasal or temporal quadrants.

INFERIOR QUADRANTS

Lymphoma

Several observers have suggested that lymphoma of the inferior orbit may feel slightly different than lymphoma of the superior quadrant. Superiorly the tumor may feel rounded, whereas inferiorly it can feel knotted and nodular. This difference in palpation characteristics is by no means diagnostic.

RISE IN BLOOD PRESSURE

There are two very unusual situations that may be encountered on palpation. Both metastatic carcinoid tumors and extra-adrenal pheochromocytomas can give rise to significant elevations of blood pressure when palpated. Systolic blood pressure may exceed 200 mm Hg. This is in contrast to patients who respond to palpation of a painful orbital tumor by elevation in blood pressure secondary to pain and anxiety or who experience a drop in blood pressure secondary to a vasovagal episode.

6
The Six P's of Orbital
Clinical Evaluation: Pulsation

The fifth "P" of orbital disease is represented by pulsation. We are reminded to not only observe and palpate the orbit, but to auscultate as well.

Orbital pulsation is generally a sign of arteriovenous malformation or of a defect in the orbital roof. Pulsation should be sought as part of a routine orbital examination by watching globe position from the front and side of the patient. Orbital pulsation can often be appreciated during slit lamp examination, especially when applanation pressures are taken. Pulsations can also be observed in the mirror of the exophthalmometer or when the patient is viewed from a lateral position.

Bruits are best heard with a bell stethoscope over a closed eyelid. The patient is asked to close both eyes, the bell stethoscope is placed on the eyelid to be examined, and the patient is asked to gently open the opposite eye to relax the orbicularis muscles. One should always hear background orbital "noise." If no background noise is heard, the maneuver is repeated with less pressure placed on the orbit by the stethoscope.

PULSATION WITHOUT BRUITS

Neurofibromatosis

Deficient development of the bones of the orbital roof and apex will often allow cerebral pulsations to be transmitted to the orbit, resulting in pulsating enophthalmos. Pulsating exophthalmos occurs if there is an associated orbital tumor. A bruit is not usually heard.

Postsurgical Pulsation

Patients who have undergone orbital surgery through a craniotomy approach may also be left with a defective bony orbital roof. Repair of the bony defect with exogenous material, such as wire mesh, can prevent this surgical complication.

Encephaloceles

Congenital dehiscences of the orbital bones may allow meninges and brain to prolapse. These are usually midline defects but can give rise to orbital pulsations if the dehiscence is sufficiently large.

Hydrocephalus

Severe, long-standing hydrocephalus can produce bony defects early in life and lead to orbital pulsation. This is a rare occurrence, however.

Metastatic Orbital Tumors

Extremely vascular orbital metastases may infrequently give rise to pulsations.

Trauma

Cranial or sinus trauma with resultant bony defects may result in transmitted orbital pulsations.

BRUITS WITH OR WITHOUT PULSATION

Arteriovenous Malformation (AVM)

Included in this category are orbital AVMs, carotid-cavernous sinus fistulas, and "lower-grade" dural AVMs (anastomoses between meningeal branches of the carotid arteries and dural veins). Pulsating proptosis may be bilateral or unilateral. Pulsation and bruit may be appreciated only on the *contralateral* side of the fistula if the ipsilateral orbital veins become thrombosed.

7
The Six P's of Orbital Clinical Evaluation: Periocular and Ocular Changes

The sixth "P" of orbital disease draws our attention from the orbit to the eye and the adnexa oculi (periorbital structures) for additional information to support our orbital diagnosis.

This aspect of orbital physical diagnosis has been largely ignored by ophthalmologists. One must be prepared to examine the periorbital tissue, including the nose, sinuses, nasopharynx, mouth, ears, lymph nodes of the neck, and in some circumstances, the entire body. The periorbital examination may lead to an "on-the-spot" diagnosis. In other cases, the periorbital changes can enable the physician to categorize a patient into a diagnostic grouping such as "vascular anomaly." It is always wise to examine the face as a whole and note the integration and relationships of various facial features. Resist the temptation of concentrating on an obviously proptotic eye. Don't miss the forest for the trees!

Salmon-Colored Mass in the Superior Cul-de-Sac

This is a characteristic sign of lymphoma when it occurs in the superior rather than the inferior orbit. The growth is subconjunctival, although an orbital component is usually present. Prominent conjunctival vessels on the surface of the tumor are also characteristic (Fig. 7-1).

Lid Retraction and Lid Lag

These are well-known hallmarks of thyroid ophthalmopathy. Lid retraction makes any underlying proptosis appear much worse and can lead to severe exposure keratitis. Upper-lid retraction probably results, at least in part, from sympathetic overstimulation of palpebral smooth muscle (Muller's muscle) and the levator palpebrae muscle. Retraction of the lower lid also occurs as smooth muscle is found in the lower eyelid in an analogous arrangement to the upper lid (Fig. 7-2). Most retractions of the lower lid, however, are probably due to fibrosis of the inferior rectus, with contracture of the attached lower lid retractors.

Pseudo Retraction of the Lid

One can be easily fooled into labeling a patient as having a thyroid condition when he or she has an apparent proptosis with pseudo-retraction of the lid. This can occur with a superior cul-de-sac lymphoma, with large filtering blebs, and when *contralateral ptosis* exists. With unilateral ptosis, Hering's law of equal innervation will produce pseudoretraction of the lid on the opposite side in an attempt to raise the ptotic lid. Mechanical elevation (with a finger) of the ptotic lid or patching of the ptotic eye will decrease the bilateral levator innervation and reverse the pseudoretraction. Overaction of the superior rectus muscle acting against a restricted inferior rectus muscle may also simulate upper-eyelid retraction.

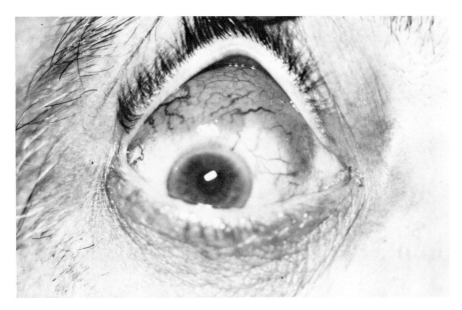

Fig. 7-1. Subconjunctival mass in the superior cul-de-sac with orbital lymphoma.

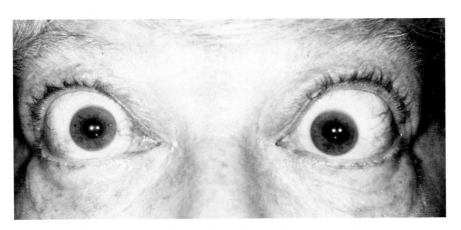

Fig. 7-2. Marked lid retraction with thyroid ophthalmopathy.

Injection Over the Lateral Rectus Muscle

A single dilated vessel (often tortuous) with small vessel injection isolated to the lateral rectus muscle is highly characteristic of thyroid eye disease (Fig. 7-3). This contrasts with the diffuse or quadrantic injection seen in pseudotumor, orbital abscess, carotid cavernous sinus fistulas, and episcleritis.

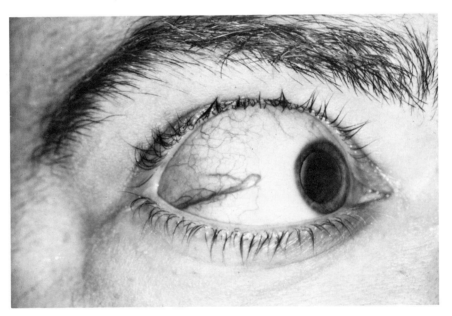

Fig. 7-3. Dilated blood vessel over the lateral rectus muscle in thyroid ophthalmopathy.

Epibulbar Corkscrew Vessels

A diffuse dilatation of the epibulbar veins with tortuosity (corkscrew configuration) extending to the limbus suggests an arteriovenous malformation (Fig. 7-4). These vessels are often dark-red, as contrasted with the purple color of the vessels in thyroid eye disease. Inflammatory pseudotumor, thrombophlebitis, and orbital abscess can also present with tortuous, dilated vessels. The surrounding conjunctival and episcleral tissue is usually injected in these cases. This contrasts with the white sclera often seen in patients with fistulas.

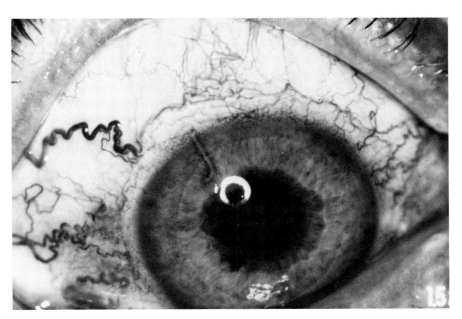

Fig. 7-4. Dilatation and tortuosity of the episcleral vessels with an arteriovenous malformation. The adjacent sclera remains white.

Extraorbital Hemangiomas

Patients with capillary hemangiomas of the orbit may also have hemangiomas of the skin (strawberry marks) elsewhere on the body (Fig. 7-5). Extraorbital hemangiomas may be found on the trunk, extremities, palate, or in the subglottic space. The subglottic tumors can lead to respiratory distress. Some patients have multiple hemangiomas involving the eye and entire body. Thrombocytopenia may be a concomitant finding in patients with capillary hemangiomas (Kasabach-Merrit syndrome).

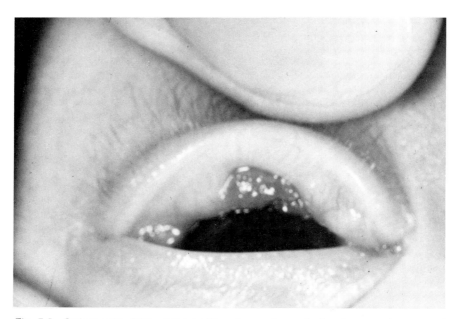

Fig. 7-5. Patient with right orbital capillary hemangioma. A strawberry mark was noted when the right upper lid was everted.

Cutaneous Vascular Anomalies

Dilated, bluish vascular anomalies on the conjunctiva, lids, scalp, and palate may occur with orbital varices or lymphangiomas. These two lesions are essentially indistinguishable from a clinical point of view (Fig. 7-6).

S-shaped Upper Eyelid

Plexiform neurofibromas may cause drooping of the lateral half of the eyelid. This produces a "sine wave" appearance that, when exaggerated, gives an S-shaped curvature to the eyelid. The disease is usually so extensive that the entire eyelid becomes hypertrophied and thickened. Other superior lateral orbital masses, such as lacrimal gland tumors, may also cause an S-shaped configuration of the upper eyelid.

Anterior Uveitis

The presence of an orbital mass and anterior uveitis should alert the physician to the possibility of sarcoidosis or orbital pseudotumor. The latter association is more common in children.

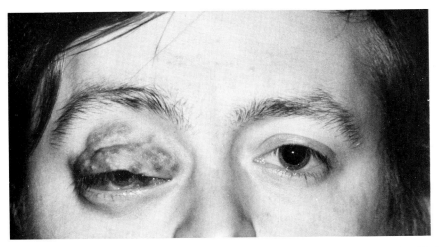

Fig. 7-6. Dilated vessels in the right upper eyelid and conjunctiva in a patient with orbital varices.

Posterior Uveitis

One must be alert to the possibility of inflammatory orbital disease such as sarcoidosis in cases of posterior uveitis. Fluffy exudates may be seen in the inferior vitreous cavity, the so-called "string of pearls" sign (Fig. 7-7). Histiocytic lymphoma (reticulum cell sarcoma) can also produce posterior uveitis.

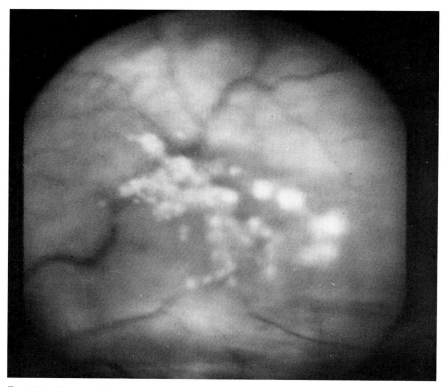

Fig. 7-7. "Snowball" exudates in the inferior vitreous cavity ("string of pearls" sign) in a patient with granulomatous invasion of the orbit.

Eczematous Lesions of the Eyelids

Patients with long-standing mycosis fungoides may occasionally develop posterior orbital involvement with proptosis and visual loss. Lid involvement is more common than deep orbital involvement (Fig. 7-8). The diagnosis is usually established by the time the orbit is involved. The eczematous and indurated cutaneous plaques characteristic of this disease are apparent on clinical examination.

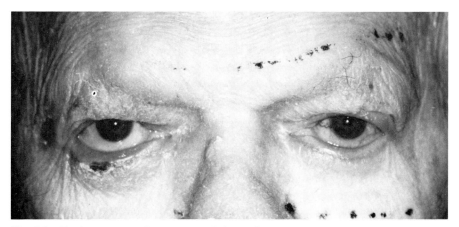

Fig. 7-8. Erythematous and eczematous lesions of the eyelids. The patient had bilateral orbital involvement with mycosis fungoides.

Molluscum Fibrosum

Multiple neurofibromas of the skin should always alert the physician to the possibility of neurofibromatosis with its associated tumors (Fig. 7-9). Other signs of neurofibromatosis include multiple café-au-lait spots, diffuse hypertrophy of the skin and subcutaneous tissues, and orbital pulsation.

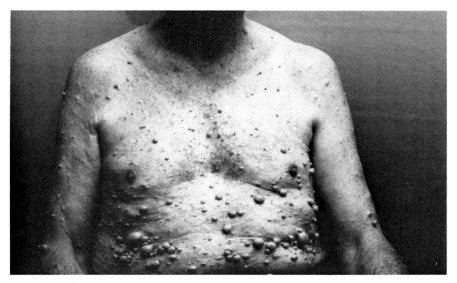

Fig. 7-9. Multiple neurocutaneous tumors with neurofibromatosis.

Conjunctival Yellowish, Fleshy Mass

The presence of this mass on the superiotemporal aspect of the globe is highly suggestive of a dermolipoma. Such a lesion often extends posteriorly into the orbit making complete surgical excision unwise because of potential secondary complications such as ptosis and symblepharon.

Eyelid Ecchymosis

True eyelid ecchymosis should lead one to suspect an orbital hemorrhage (traumatic or spontaneous), neuroblastoma (Racoon sign), or leukemia (granulocytic sarcoma) (Fig. 7-10). The latter two are often bilateral but not necessarily simultaneous.

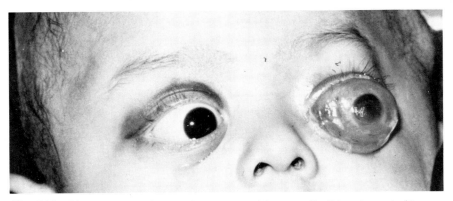

Fig. 7-10. Bilateral proptosis secondary to neuroblastoma. Eyelid ecchymosis (Racoon sign) is present.

Fullness over Temporalis Muscle

Patients with sphenoid wing meningiomas can develop fullness of the temporalis muscle fossa secondary to outward tumor invasion (Fig. 7-11). This may also be seen with metastatic tumors and advanced malignant lacrimal gland tumors.

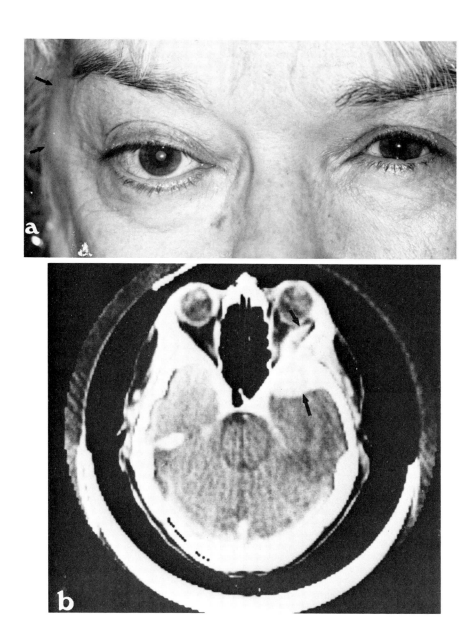

Fig. 7-11. (A) Bulging of the temporalis muscle fossa (arrows). (B) Computed tomography reveals invasive sphenoid wing meningioma (arrows).

Swelling of Lateral Lower Lid

Edema of the eyelids may be associated with large orbital apex meningiomas. This is a curious, uncommon sign of meningioma and has not been satisfactorily explained to date. The edema usually occurs with longstanding meningiomas and is not associated with inflammatory signs (Fig. 7-12).

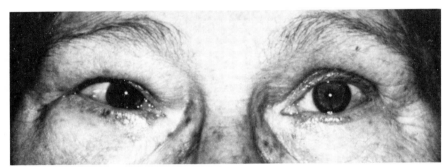

Fig. 7-12. Swelling of the right lower eyelid with an orbital apex meningioma.

Optic Nerve Dysplasia

The presence of an anomalous disc should lead one to suspect an encephalocele, especially when there is a midline mass present (Fig. 7-13). *All* nasal and nasopharyngeal masses associated with an anomalous disc should be treated as encephaloceles. Appropriate radiographic studies should be carried out before any such mass is biopsied or excised. Failure to examine the disc carefully and suspect this diagnosis has made many an orbital surgeon "neurosurgeon for a day."

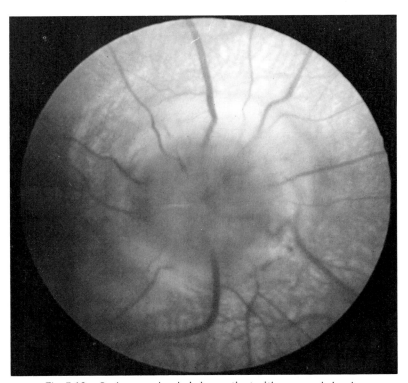

Fig. 7-13. Optic nerve dysplasia in a patient with an encephalocele.

Opticociliary Shunt Vessels

Any compressive optic nerve lesion can produce opticociliary shunt vessels (Fig. 7-14). The tumor most commonly associated with these anomalous vessels is the optic nerve sheath meningioma. Other tumors to be considered include gliomas, sphenoid wing meningiomas invading the orbit, and rarely, optic nerve sarcoidosis. They may be seen with bony compression, such as in craniosynostosis. Shunt vessels have also been noted following central retinal vein occlusion, chronic papilledema, and as a congenital variant. The shunt vessels represent dilatation of preexisting surface vessels that drain into the choroidal venous system.

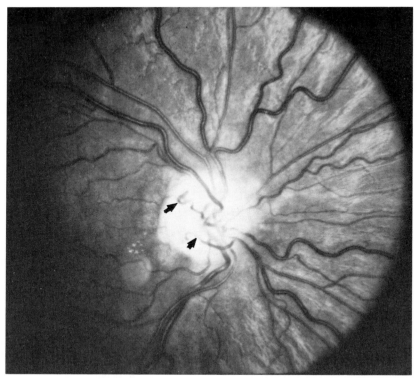

Fig. 7-14. Opticociliary shunt vessels (arrows) secondary to an optic nerve sheath meningioma.

Choroidal Folds, Scleral Indentation

Past authors have considered choroidal folds to be a reliable sign of orbital tumors (Fig. 7-15). It was felt that one could localize the tumor's position by careful observation of the choroidal pattern. It is now clear that choroidal folds are a nonspecific finding encountered in a number of conditions. Choroidal folds secondary to orbital tumors do not necessarily correspond to the tumor's location and do not necessarily imply pressure on the globe by the tumor. They can be seen with a diffuse increase in orbital pressure, such as in thyroid ophthalmopathy. They can also occur with papilledema and ocular hypotony, and they are occasionally idiopathic. Visual field defects (especially temporal) can be produced. The folds may persist for many years following resection of the inciting orbital tumor. Many orbital tumors will produce a smooth indentation of the sclera rather than choroidal folds.

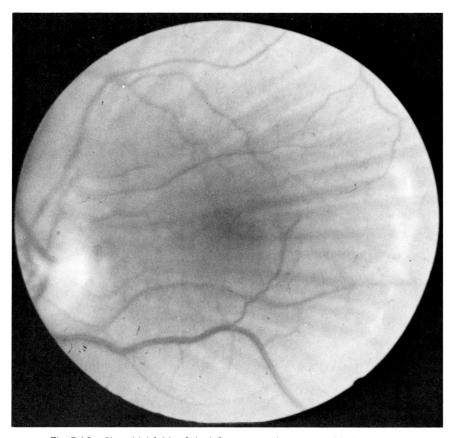

Fig. 7-15. Choroidal folds of the left eye secondary to an orbital mass lesion.

Frozen Globe

Acute or subacute proptosis with marked limitation of motility should lead one to suspect metastatic disease or a fungal infection such as mucormycosis. Other conditions to be considered include orbital cellulitis, venous thrombosis secondary to cellulitis or an arteriovenous fistula, and inflammatory orbital pseudotumor.

Black Crusted Lesions of the Palate

An orbital examination is never complete without an examination of the nose and paranasal structures. One must always examine these structures when dealing with a "frozen globe" or any combination of proptosis and ophthalmoplegia. The presence of diabetes or an immunosuppressed condition should alert one to the possibility of phycomycosis. The two organisms most commonly identified in this condition are *Mucor* and *Rhizopus*. One will often see the black palatal eschar early in the course of the disease (Fig. 7-16). All atypical cases of orbital cellulitis or cavernous sinus thrombosis should be inspected daily for this dismal sign. The lesions represent areas of infarction and necrosis secondary to arterial invasion by the fungus.

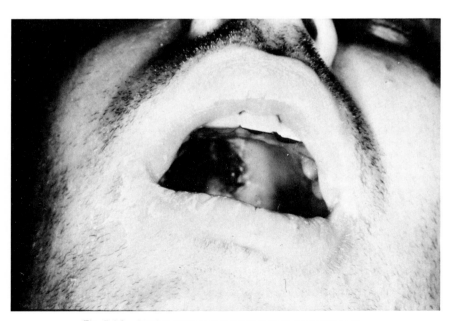

Fig. 7-16. Black palatal eschar secondary to mucormycosis.

Facial Asymmetry

Progressive facial asymmetry is seen in neurofibromatosis, fibrous dysplasia, and the Parry-Romberg syndrome. Other less severe forms are seen in tuberous sclerosis, the Sturge-Weber syndrome, and with large osteomas. Parry-Romberg syndrome or progressive facial hemiatrophy often produces enophthalmos, thinning of the skin, bone atrophy, and loss of eyelashes. Pupillary abnormalities, including Horner's syndrome, are often noted. In contrast, patients with neurofibromatosis can have facial hemihypertrophy rather than atrophy, and the skin is usually redundant rather than thinned.

Fibrous dysplasia can produce distortion and abnormal calcification of the orbital bones. The patients usually note facial asymmetry with painless swelling over the involved bones in the second decade of life. Proptosis is common, and there is often some downward displacement of the globe as well. More posterior orbital involvement can produce optic atrophy.

Abduction Blindness

Patients with optic nerve sheath meningiomas usually experience a slowly progressive decrease in central vision. Some of these patients will notice a further momentary drop in acuity when they abduct the involved eye. The pupil of the involved eye may dilate briskly, and retinal arteriolar pulsations may be seen. Acuity returns to its baseline level when the eye is returned to primary position.

Oculodigital Sign

Infants and young children with severe visual dysfunction may periodically press on the affected eye with their fingers. This has been noted in various ocular diseases and may be a mechanical attempt to produce phosphenes. This sign may also be seen in cases of reduced visual acuity secondary to capillary hemangiomas (Fig. 7-17).

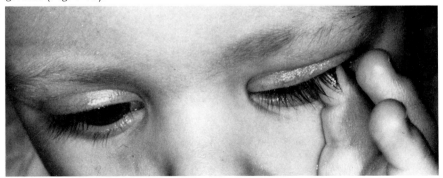

Fig. 7-17. Oculodigital sign with orbital capillary hemangioma. Visual acuity in the left eye was markedly reduced secondary to anisometropic amblyopia.

8
The Laboratory Workup

Prior to undertaking the laboratory investigation of a patient with an orbital problem, the clinician attempts to place the disease process into a broad category (i.e., vascular, inflammatory) based on history and clinical findings. This "working diagnosis" then guides the clinician toward the most appropriate diagnostic tests. The temptation to plunge into an extensive laboratory workup before utilizing all clinical information available must be avoided. One would never think of subjecting a patient with bloody stools to an upper and lower GI series without first checking carefully for hemorrhoids. Similarly, in this age of "radiation paranoia," one should never subject a patient to expensive, time-consuming procedures until a tentative clinical diagnosis has been reached. As tests are completed and further information is obtained, the "working diagnosis," and thus the emphasis of the investigation, may change.

Over-reliance on computed tomography (CT scan) may lead to unnecessary surgical explorations and incorrect surgical approaches, with resultant morbidity and mortality. The most striking example of this is seen in patients with thyroid eye disease. The enlarged muscles associated with this disease have often been mistaken for orbital tumors (Fig. 8-1). Many patients have been subjected to lateral orbitotomies and craniotomies in search of a mass that only existed on a computer printout. Close attention to the history and physical examination and confidence in one's clinical judgment will prevent many of these errors.

Good clinical judgment is aided by a knowledge of the relative incidence of various orbital diseases. With few exceptions (such as Burkitt's lymphoma in Africa), the incidence of orbital tumors is rather constant in all parts of the world. The incidences of various orbital diseases an ophthalmologist might expect to see have been previously outlined (see Chapter 1). Common diseases

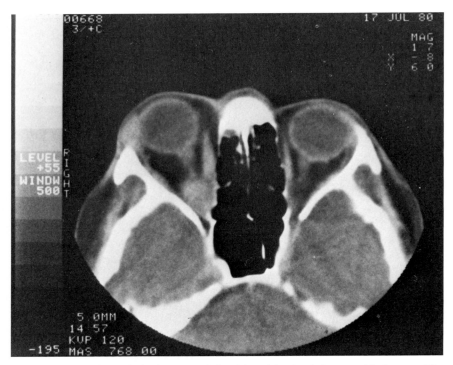

Fig. 8-1. Enlarged muscle in the apex of the right orbit, simulating an orbital tumor. The medial rectus muscle is also thickened.

such as thyroid ophthalmopathy may present in an atypical fashion. Therefore, the more common diseases should always be considered and ruled out before an esoteric diagnosis is entertained. When you hear hoofbeats, look first for horses, *then* for unicorns!

Figure 8-2 outlines a logical progression of laboratory testing that one might follow in the evaluation of patients with orbital disease. The "shotgun" approach to laboratory diagnosis must be avoided.

Patients identified as having thyroid eye disease on clinical examination are evaluated by an internist or endocrinologist. Chemical diagnosis of thyroid abnormality involves T3, T4, and TSH (thyroid-stimulating hormone) determinations. This is usually sufficient when the clinical findings, ultrasound, and/or CT scan are typical for the disease. However, when these blood studies are nondiagnostic, further laboratory testing may be necessary. More-sensitive tests of thyroid dysfunction include the TRH stimulation test, and the Werner T3 suppression test. Stimulation of TSH by TRH (thyroid-releasing hormone) has become the most valuable of the two and can detect an abnormality in approximately 75 percent of patients with thyroid ophthalmopathy. This test

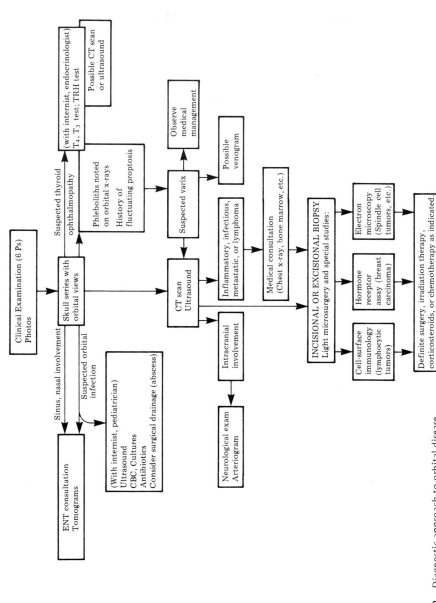

Fig. 8-2. Diagnostic approach to orbital disease.

65

is rapidly replacing T3 suppression, which is more difficult to perform and has been associated with serious side effects such as cardiac arrythmias. Chemically euthyroid patients should be followed closely with serum T4 and T3 levels repeated at regular intervals. Most patients will be found to have abnormal thyroid function studies sometime in the course of their disease. It must be stressed that a normal T4, T3, or TSH does not rule out thyroid ophthalmopathy. The clinical ophthalmic findings are sensitive and reliable indicators of thyroid dysfunction. Chemical corroboration is not essential in the diagnosis of thyroid eye disease.

Patients with bilateral findings classic of thyroid eye disease (such as lid retraction) and overt systemic thyroid hormonal imbalance may not require further orbital evaluation. Patients with unilateral proptosis or any atypical features should have an orbital ultrasound and/or CT scan to confirm the diagnosis of thyroid eye disease. Both may be necessary in difficult cases.

As an adjunct to clinical examination, patients should be photographed. This is a valuable aid in patient follow-up and is a most accurate method of documentation. Patients occasionally may need to be reminded visually that their lid was ptotic before surgery and not as a result of it.

RADIOLOGIC STUDIES

Skull X-rays

Skull and orbital x-rays can provide data regarding the nature, extent, and operability of an orbital disease process. They are an integral part of the orbital workup and an important diagnostic step after completion of the physical examination. Skull x-rays with orbital views are obtained in most patients with orbital disease *before* computed tomography. The skull films, in conjunction with the history and physical, will help determine the type of further studies to be ordered and may eliminate the need for more studies altogether. For example, the presence of phleboliths (usually secondary to varices) on skull x-ray may indicate the need for venography rather than for CT scan. An opacified sinus on skull series would mandate special sinus views not ordinarily obtainable with an orbit or brain CT scan. Additionally, one might obtain an ENT evaluation and conventional tomography before a CT scan if sinus disease were present. In addition to sinus views, one should also obtain optic foramen views, especially in patients with visual loss.

Lacrimal Gland Fossa Changes

The plain skull x-ray remains a most valuable modality for evaluating the lacrimal gland fossa. The common lesions encountered are inflammatory pseudotumor, lymphoma, benign and malignant epithelial tumors, and dermoid cysts.

Skull x-rays are usually normal with lymphoma and pseudotumor. One will frequently see pressure enlargement of the lacrimal gland fossa without destruction of bone with benign mixed lacrimal gland tumors (pleomorphic adenomas) (Fig. 8-3). With malignant epithelial tumors, the x-rays will be negative or show fossa enlargement in about half the cases. The remaining cases will display either bone destruction, sclerosis, or calcification in the lacrimal gland fossa.

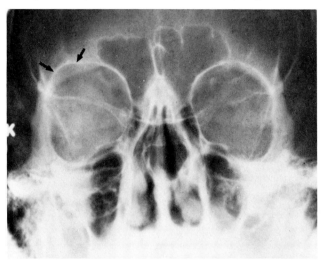

Fig. 8-3. Pressure enlargement of the right lacrimal gland fossa on plain skull x-rays (arrows).

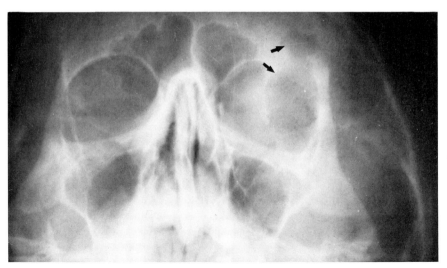

Fig. 8-4. Left-sided orbital dermoid producing bony defects in the superior orbit and adjacent frontal bone (arrows).

Dermoid cysts often produce cystic defects along the superior bony rim of the orbit (Fig. 8-4). "Egg shell" calcifications in the walls of the cyst are seen in chronic cases.

Less-common lacrimal gland fossa lesions such as plasmacytoma and metastatic tumors will often produce bone destruction. Osteoblastic lesions may be seen with prostatic and breast metastases. In summary, lacrimal gland fossa tumors that cause bone changes include (1) benign mixed tumor (pleomorphic adenoma), (2) malignant epithelial lacrimal gland tumor, (3) dermoid cyst, (4) plasmacytoma, and (5) metastatic tumor.

Sinus Changes

Opacification of the sinus is an early sign of sinusitis. The presence of an · air fluid level can help differentiate sinusitis from hemorrhage or neoplasms. Chronic sinusitis leads to thickened mucosa and proliferative osteitis. Associated

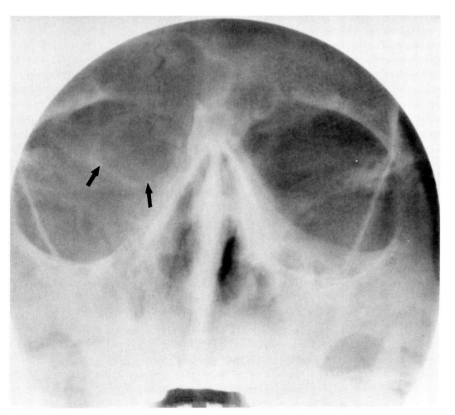

Fig. 8-5. Downward expansion of the superior orbital roof with a frontal sinus mucocele (arrows).

conditions include cellulitis, abscess formation, and occasionally a granuloma-tous or inflammatory (pseudotumor) orbital response. Osteomyelitis may be a serious life-threatening sequel.

Expansion of the frontal sinus with downward displacement of the supraorbi-tal ridge is a characteristic sign of mucoceles (Fig. 8-5). The sinus is usually opaque, but extensive bone destruction can produce a radiolucent or normal appearance. The margins of the sinus may be rounded, thickened, or show evidence of destruction. Differential diagnosis includes inverted papilloma, retention cyst, or carcinoma.

Ethmoidal mucoceles may be difficult to identify on skull x-rays. Nonspecific findings include destruction of ethmoidal septa, loss of ethmoidal cell trans-lucency, and lateral expansion of the medial orbital rim. There is often concom-itant involvement of the sphenoid sinus, which is easier to identify radiographi-cally. With sphenoid sinus mucoceles, opacification may be associated with expansion of the sinus, destruction of the floor of the pituitary fossa, and erosion of the optic canal medially. Differential diagnosis includes neoplasms, carotid artery aneurysms, and pituitary tumors.

Osteomas are slow-growing tumors that present radiographically as round, well-demarcated opacities most commonly occurring in the frontal and eth-moidal sinuses. They are often incidental findings on routine skull x-rays (Fig. 8-6). More aggressive tumors can produce proptosis, globe displacement, and facial asymmetry (Fig. 8-7).

Sinus opacification with bony destruction is a frequent finding with malig-nant sinus tumors. Squamous cell carcinoma is the most common tumor encoun-tered. The maxillary sinus is most frequently involved.

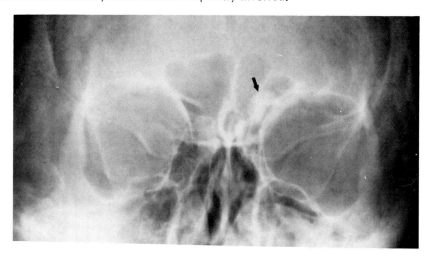

Fig. 8-6. Asymptomatic osteoma in the left frontal sinus (arrow).

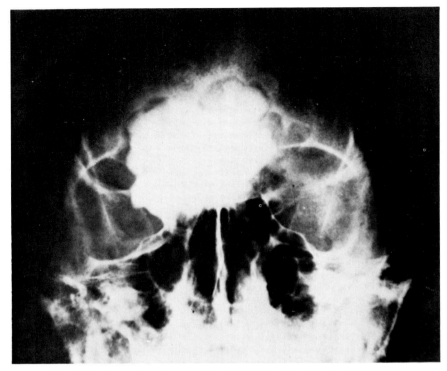

Fig. 8-7. Aggressive osteoma of the frontal sinus invading the right orbit.

Optic Canal Changes

The anterior aspect of the optic canal (foramen) is demonstrated by plain x-rays. Tomographic studies are required when one wishes to view the entire length of the optic canal. Enlargement of the optic foramen is diagnosed by comparison with the other side, not solely by absolute measurements. There is considerable variation in the size of optic foramina, but generally a difference greater than 1.5 mm is considered abnormal. Optic canals reach their full size at about age 5. A foramen greater than 7 mm in diameter should be regarded as highly suspicious. Measurements taken in the horizontal plane are more reliable than vertical measurements. Congenital variations can produce elongation of the canal in the vertical meridian, which may be misleading.

Optic foramen enlargement may be caused by optic nerve glioma, neurofibromatosis with arachnoidal hyperplasia, optic nerve meningioma, invasive retinoblastoma, optic nerve granuloma, or ophthalmic artery aneurysm.

Glioma is the most common cause of optic canal enlargement (Fig. 8-8). Arachnoidal hyperplasia beyond the extent of a glioma or in association with neurofibromatosis may enlarge the canal, but this is uncommon. Meningiomas

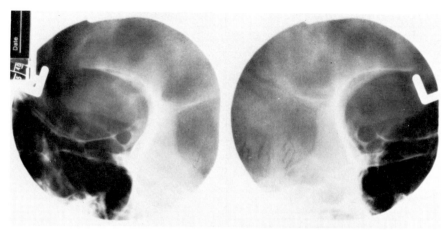

Fig. 8-8. Optic canal enlargement on the left side with optic nerve glioma.

can cause enlargement of the canal, but hyperostosis or erosion is more common. Optic nerve invasion by retinoblastoma is usually an obvious diagnosis based on history or eye examination. Optic nerve granulomas may be idiopathic or secondary to sarcoidosis or aspergillosis. Aneurysms of the ophthalmic artery are uncommon but can cause progressive monocular visual loss. Arteriography is usually required for diagnosis.

Other less-common causes of optic canal enlargement include infections or malignancies of the sphenoid bone and anterior extension of parasellar tumors such as craniopharyngioma.

Causes of optic foramen erosion include meningioma (see above), metastatic lesions, sphenoidal–ethmoidal disease, optic nerve granulomas (see above), and ophthalmic artery aneurysm (see above).

The optic foramen may appear smaller on the side of the lesion secondary to hyperostosis. Optic canal hyperostosis can be caused by fibrous dysplasia, osteopetrosis, or meningioma.

Superior Orbital Fissure Changes

Superior orbital fissure changes may be due to carotid aneurysm, isolated neurofibroma, arteriovenous fistulas, plasmacytoma, meningioma, hemangiopericytoma, granulomatous disease, sinus or nasopharyngeal tumor, neurofibromatosis (posterior encephalocele), or pituitary adenoma.

The superior orbital fissure can usually be seen on plain orbital views. An infraclinoid or intracavernous aneurysm is probably the most common cause of fissure widening. Isolated neurofibromas can arise from branches of the nasociliary nerve and cause fissure enlargement. Several other lesions, such as inflammatory pseudotumor and lymphoma, have been reported to produce changes in the superior orbital fissure. These cases are most unusual, however.

Orbital Calcification

Ocular calcifications can occur with retinoblastoma, retrolental fibroplasia, and phthisis bulbi. Orbital conditions producing calcification include:

1. Venous malformations—Phleboliths are associated with vascular abnormalities such as varices
2. Malignant lacrimal gland tumors—Calcification has been reported in a small percentage of patients with malignant lacrimal gland fossa tumors
3. Optic nerve sheath meningiomas (less common)
4. Dermoid cysts (less common)
5. Hemangioma (less common)

Computed tomography may be helpful in the detection of orbital calcifications (Fig. 8-9).

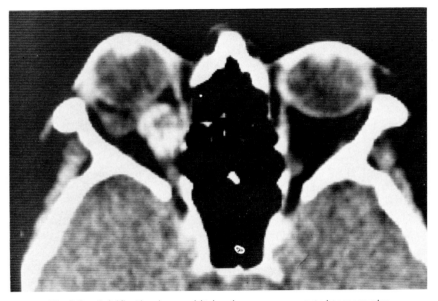

Fig. 8-9. Calcification in an orbital varix seen on computed tomography.

Increased and Decreased Orbital Size

Any long-standing orbital tumor, especially in childhood, may produce orbital enlargement. Vascular anomalies and slow-growing primary tumors of the orbit probably constitute the leading causes of generalized orbital enlargement. Other causes of orbital enlargement include congenital glaucoma with buphthalmus, neurofibromatosis, and meningoencephaloceles.

Decreased orbital size is usually seen following enucleation. Orbital irradiation in infancy or early childhood may also decrease orbital size. Other causes include phthisis bulbi, anophthalmos, microphthalmos, craniosynostosis, fibrous dysplasia, Paget's disease, Apert's syndrome, osteogenesis imperfecta, and surgical orbitotomy in childhood. Bone removal is usually unnecessary when performing an orbitotomy on a child and can result in significant facial deformity.

Sphenoid Hyperostosis

Sphenoid wing meningiomas may produce hyperostosis of the lesser wing of the sphenoid (Fig. 8-10). Any increase in orbital density from tumor, edema, or inflammation can produce a decrease in orbital translucence. The lesser wing of the sphenoid may, therefore, appear to be more dense. This "pseudo-hyperostosis" may be falsely interpreted as a sign of meningioma or osteoblastic metastases. Similarly, "pseudo-hyperostosis" may be noted if the head is rotated when posterior-anterior skull films are taken. True hyperostosis of the sphenoid can be confirmed by conventional tomography.

Loss of the oblique orbital line (innominate line) usually signals invasion of the outer sphenoid by a malignant tumor or meningioma (Fig. 8-11). An enlarged sphenoid sinus (pneumosinus dilatans) may indicate the presence of an adjacent meningioma.

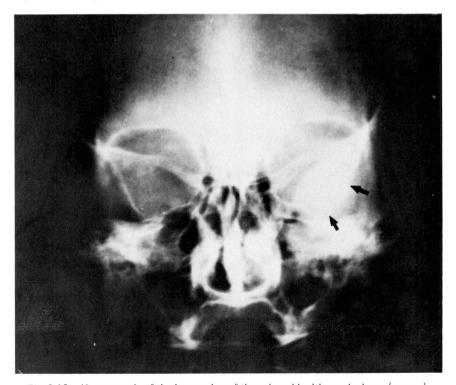

Fig. 8-10. Hyperostosis of the lesser wing of the sphenoid with meningioma (arrows).

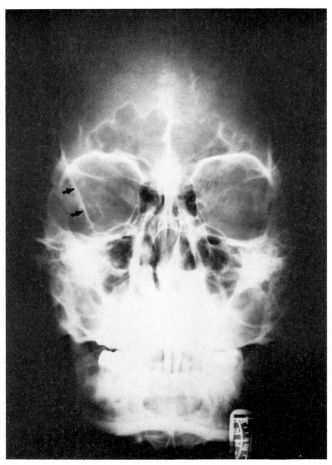

Fig. 8-11. Loss of the innominate line of the left orbit secondary to an invasive meningioma. The right innominate line is present (arrows).

Conventional Tomography

Computed tomography (axial and coronal) has largely replaced conventional tomography in the evaluation of soft tissue abnormalities of the orbit. Further refinements in CT scanning have reduced (but not eliminated) the need for conventional tomography in other situations, and this trend will no doubt continue.

Conventional tomography remains a valuable aid in the evaluation of optic canal changes, bone changes on plain x-ray, trauma, the paranasal sinuses, and lacrimal gland fossa changes. Hypocycloidal polytomography is the preferred mode of conventional tomography.

Optic Canal Changes

Basal tomography is a most useful technique for visualizing both canals on a single radiograph, allowing comparison of both sides (Fig. 8-12). Axial or coronal tomography of each canal can also be performed. Intracanalicular or intracranial involvement by optic nerve tumors such as optic nerve meningiomas may not be demonstrated by axial CT scanning alone. Conventional tomography may show up an abnormality early in the course of these tumors and should be considered in the workup of unexplained, progressive, visual loss. Intracranial involvement will occasionally occur in the absence of any radiologic change.

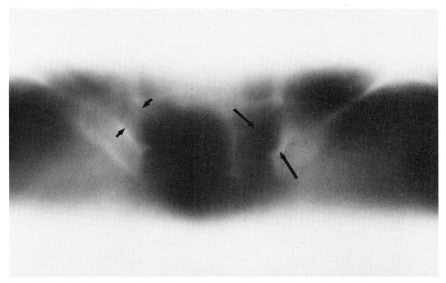

Fig. 8-12. Basal tomography of the optic canals. The right optic canal is normal (short arrows). The left optic canal is enlarged. The margins are eroded and ill-defined (long arrows).

Bone Change on Plain X-ray

Investigation by conventional tomography should be considered when destruction, hyperostosis, or indentation of the bony orbital walls is demonstrated on plain x-rays. Both axial and coronal tomography can be helpful in evaluating the orbital apex. Osseous tumors should also be evaluated with conventional tomography. Multiple tomographic cuts can be helpful in delineating the extent of tumor growth.

Trauma

Conventional tomography will frequently detect orbital wall fractures not readily seen on plain films or CT scanning. Tomograms are useful in the evaluation of suspected orbital floor fractures and optic canal fractures, in which a combination of coronal and axial views can be employed. Lateral tomography can be useful in determining the posterior extent of blow-out fractures and frontal sinus mucoceles.

The Paranasal Sinuses

Axial tomography can be especially helpful in evaluation of the ethmoidal and sphenoid sinuses.

Lacrimal Gland Fossa Changes

The plain x-ray is invaluable in the evaluation of tumors in this area. Occasionally, one will see subtle characteristic changes on tomography (coronal, lateral) that are not appreciated on plain films alone.

ORBITAL VENOGRAPHY

This technique has been replaced in most centers by CT scanning and ultrasound. The technique necessitates a venipuncture into a frontal or angular vein and injection of contrast material. The superior ophthalmic vein is then visualized, and information is obtained by noting displacement, obstruction,

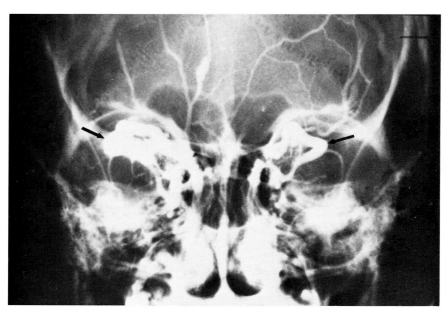

Fig. 8-13. Bilateral orbital varices with diffuse dilatation of the superior ophthalmic veins (arrows).

or dilatation of the venous system. Information obtained in many centers is less than optimal, as fewer radiologists are now being trained in this technique.

Venography is reserved for difficult diagnostic cases of orbital vascular abnormalities. The venographic findings in orbital varices include focal saccular dilatations of the veins or diffuse dilatation throughout the orbit (Fig. 8-13). The presence of an arteriovenous fistula may also be suggested by failure to fill the venous system because of backflow pressure.

Venography may also be occasionally indicated in the evaluation of the cavernous sinus. Expert radiologic consultation is again essential to make the test worthwhile. Obstruction of the vein in the cavernous sinus can indicate the presence of granulomatous tissue such as seen in the Tolosa-Hunt syndrome. This is not a specific finding, however, and any mass lesion, such as a meningioma, can produce a similar picture.

ORBITAL ARTERIOGRAPHY

Arteriography of the orbit is useful in the preoperative evaluation of orbital masses that extend into the cranial vault or intracranial lesions that extend into the orbit.

Arteriography can also be useful in the evaluation of arteriovenous fistulas, secondary orbital varices, hemangiopericytomas, and meningiomas. Generally, carotid arteriography is not indicated in the routine evaluation of primary orbital tumors. Even in situations of presumed cavernous hemangiomas in adults, arteriography is *not* indicated, since these lesions are probably of venous origin and have a relatively static blood flow pattern.

COMPUTED TOMOGRAPHY

Most physicians are well aware of computed tomography and its dramatic impact on modern medicine. The basic CT unit employs a source of x-rays, which are detected and evaluated after passing through the body. Analysis is done by computer, and the results are projected on a display unit. The techniques and results have been well described.

Further refinements in the scanners continue to increase the wealth of information obtained. The progression from first generation to subsequent generation scanners has resulted in more rapid, simplified testing and higher spatial resolution. Procedures such as venography, contrast orbitography, and pneumoencephalography have largely been replaced by this technique.

CT scanning is the best available technique for *detection* and *localization* of orbital and periorbital lesions. It is indispensable in the planning of surgical approaches to the orbit. Tumors can often be localized to various anatomical compartments of the orbit. The appropriate surgical approach can then be planned to obtain optimal exposure of the orbital lesion. CT scanning is also useful in evaluating the extent of primary paranasal and nasopharyngeal masses (Fig. 8-14). Extension of an orbital lesion into the sinuses or intracranial spaces is also usually detectable. Coronal scanning allows one to further visualize the relationship of an orbital tumor to the optic nerve, extraocular muscles, and blood vessels. Optic canal changes may also be evaluated with coronal CT scanning (Fig. 8-15).

The location of a lesion (within or outside the muscle cone) and the nature of the boundaries of a lesion (smooth or irregular) can be helpful parameters in the differential diagnosis of orbital lesions. For example, the cavernous hemangioma has a smooth and regular outline and is intraconal in location. Hemangiomas are usually located between the lateral rectus muscle and the optic nerve. Lymphoma or inflammatory pseudotumor has ill-defined tissue borders and often infiltrates within and outside the muscle cone. Dermoid cysts are smooth and regular but usually are located outside the muscle cone. Orbital varices or lymphangioma are usually irregular in outline and often lie in the nasal aspect of the muscle cone between the optic nerve and medial rectus muscle.

Despite many technical advances, there are still pitfalls in the technique and diagnostic capability of computerized tomography. The CT scan does not allow good "histologic differentiation" of orbital tumors. A-scan ultrasonogra-

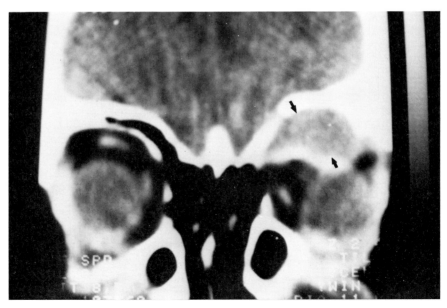

Fig. 8-14. Frontal mucocele invading the left orbit (arrows).

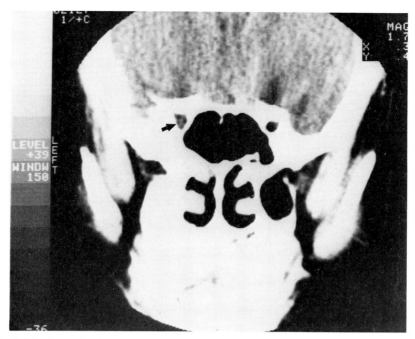

Fig. 8-15. Coronal CT scan reveals enlargement of the right optic canal (arrow). The patient was found to have sarcoidosis of the right optic nerve that invaded the chiasm.

phy is still more valuable in this regard. A CT scan may not pick up vascular abnormalities such as small varices and arteriovenous malformations.

Acute orbital abscesses may be missed on CT scan, possibly showing only diffuse signs of intraorbital inflammation such as a thickened scleral uveal rim. Orbital foreign bodies may be missed with routine CT scanning. To detect foreign bodies, one must eliminate soft tissue densities and "scatter" from the foreign bodies by adjusting the "window level" of the CT cuts. This reconstruction should be performed on the scanner monitor with a radiologist. One must not rely on CT photographs alone to rule out an orbital foreign body.

Subtle bone changes may best be evaluated by conventional tomography, which will reveal more about the character of change. The bony architecture, including margins, trabecular pattern, and presence of osteoblastic versus osteolytic change is best detected with skull films or conventional tomography at present.

It is essential to ask specifically for an "orbit scan." Evaluation of the orbit requires different positioning than a "brain scan." Contrast enhancement does not usually alter the clinical reading significantly. Therefore, contrast should not be used in patients with known or suspected reactions to iodinated contrast material.

Optic Nerve Enlargement

Enlargement of the optic nerve on CT scan is most commonly seen with gliomas or meningiomas. Other less-common causes of thickened optic nerves include optic nerve sheath cysts, inflammatory pseudotumor (Fig. 8-16), metastatic disease, granulomatous disease (sarcoid, aspergillosis), and angioma.

Remember that *conventional* basal tomography is still a useful test for determining intracranial extension of optic nerve tumors.

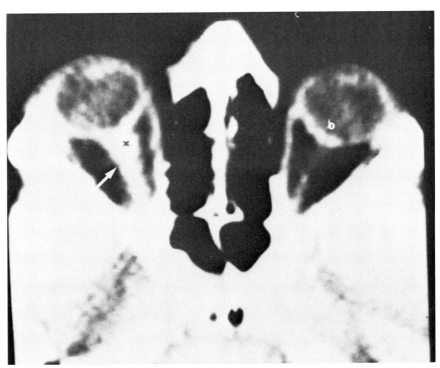

Fig. 8-16. Thickening of the right optic nerve with orbital inflammatory pseudotumor (arrow). The patient experienced pain and a marked decrease of visual acuity, which responded promptly to treatment with corticosteroids.

Thickened Extraocular Muscles

Thyroid eye disease is the most common cause of enlarged extraocular muscles. Enlargement of the superior rectus–levator complex in the orbital apex may simulate a tumor. Similarly, a fat inferior rectus can simulate a mass within the muscle cone beneath the optic nerve (Fig. 8-17). This "pseudomass" effect becomes more apparent when the muscle is contracted in at-

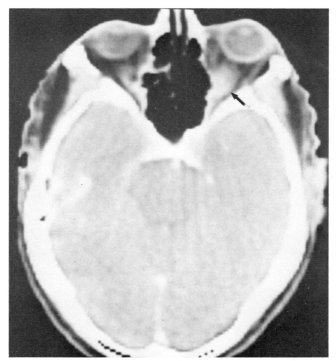

Fig. 8-17. Thickened left inferior rectus muscle with thyroid ophthalmopathy simulating an intraconal mass lesion (arrow).

tempted downgaze. To avoid this problem, the patient's eyes must be kept in primary position throughout the initial scanning. Of course, many patients with thyroid ophthalmopathy have a downward deviation of their eyes secondary to fibrosis. This compounds the problem. Coronal scanning of the muscles may also be helpful in distinguishing a tumor from an enlarged muscle (Fig. 8-18). The normal lateral rectus muscle gets wider as you move posteriorly on coronal sections. This normal finding may be misinterpreted as muscle enlargement. Thickening of the medial and lateral rectus muscles is usually obvious on axial CT scanning. The inferior rectus muscle, however, is the one most clinically affected by thyroid ophthalmopathy. The muscle insertions are usually normal in appearance and do not enhance with contrast.

The optic nerve retains its normal thickness in thyroid ophthalmopathy even when there is visual loss. Visual loss may result from compression of the optic nerve in the orbital apex by the enlarged extraocular muscles.

Arteriovenous malformations may produce a clinical picture similar to thyroid eye disease, making the diagnosis difficult. Bilateral chemosis, erythema,

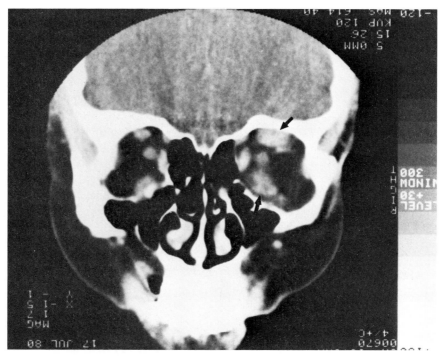

Fig. 8-18. Coronal CT scan reveals thickening of the extraocular muscles (arrows).

elevated intraocular pressure, limited motility, and ocular discomfort can all be features of both diseases. One must search carefully for an enlarged superior ophthalmic vein, a characteristic sign of fistulas (Fig. 8-19). Dilatation of this vein and the veins in the extraocular muscles occurs secondary to a rise in orbital venous pressure. Thrombosis of the superior ophthalmic vein can lead to further enlargement of the extraocular muscles as veins within the muscles dilate in a compensatory fashion.

Orbital myositis (inflammatory pseudotumor involving the extraocular muscles) often produces thickening of only one muscle and is frequently painful (Fig. 8-20). The thickened muscle will often revert to normal size after treatment with steroids. Additional findings of orbital inflammation include (1) thickening of the sclerouveal rim, which enhances with contrast; (2) diffuse infiltrating orbital mass, which may blend in with adjacent normal orbital tissue; (3) thickening of the optic nerve (perineuritis); and (4) contrast enhancement around the lacrimal gland. Metastatic disease to the extraocular muscles is occasionally seen (Fig. 8-21).

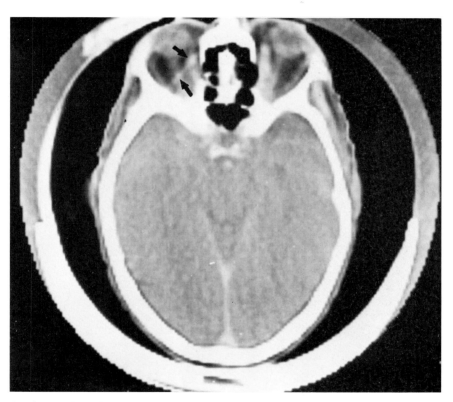

Fig. 8-19. The right superior ophthalmic vein is enlarged secondary to an arteriovenous malformation (arrows).

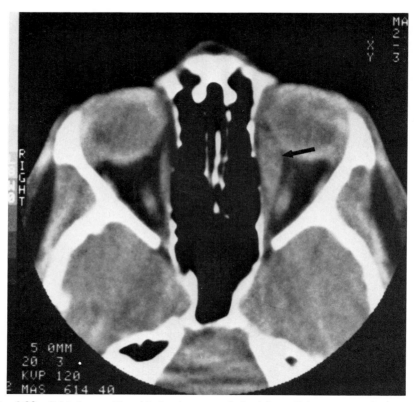

Fig. 8-20. Orbital myositis with involvement of the left medial rectus muscle (arrow). The patient's complaints of pain and diplopia were relieved within 24 hours of beginning treatment with corticosteroids.

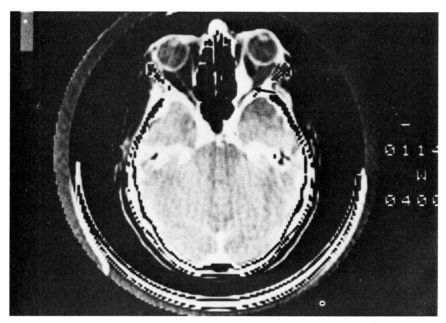

Fig. 8-21. Carcinoid tumor metastatic to the left medial rectus muscle (arrow).

"Clinical Pearls"

The following clinical points on CT scanning may prove helpful.

1. The CT scan is generally an excellent technique for evaluating intracranial spread of an orbital tumor. It is not infallible, however, especially in the orbital apex and with optic nerve tumors (Fig. 8-22).
2. Many head scanners are capable of obtaining coronal sections. However, the patient may be required to hyperextend the neck and hold it in an uncomfortable position. Most patients are incapable of doing this. It is possible, however, to get good coronal sections with a body scanner.
3. Inflammatory pseudotumor can give the appearance of a discrete orbital tumor on CT scanning. Surgical exploration will often fail to locate this "mass" because only orbital fat and surrounding connective tissue may be involved. The surgeon must be familiar with the appearance of normal orbital fat as a discoloration may be the only intraoperative evidence of an inflammatory process.
4. A dermoid tumor may have a cyst-like appearance, with a thickened wall and a relatively low-density center. In addition, one may see a layering-out of fatty oils by scanning in different head positions. This is one of the few

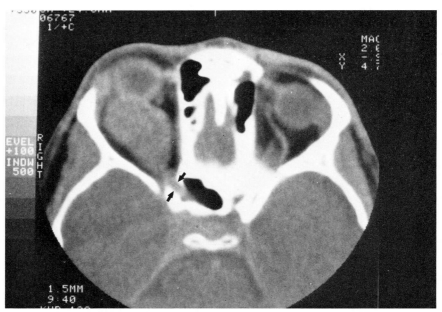

Fig. 8-22. Optic nerve glioma with thickening of the right optic nerve. The optic canal appears to be enlarged secondary to tumor invasion (arrows). The intracanalicular portion of the optic nerve was found to be normal, however, during neurosurgical exploration.

cases in which CT scanning can provide some histologic differentiation on the basis of appearance alone.

5. Subtle calcifications within tumors may be picked up with CT scanning.
6. Bone destruction is more commonly seen with malignant tumors or infections, whereas bone expansion is often associated with benign tumors.
7. There is often a space between a cavernous hemangioma and the orbital apex, which can be seen on CT scan (Fig. 4-5). This contrasts with a meningioma where the apex may be filled with tumor.

ULTRASONOGRAPHY

Ultrasound examination is an efficient, inexpensive, and safe method of evaluating the orbit and should be considered an extension of the physical examination. It is readily available to most clinicians. The two display modes used clinically are the A scan and B scan.

A-scan displays are projected along a horizontal baseline. Vertical deflections or echo spikes are dependent on the size, shape, consistency, and vascularity of the tumor. Therefore, A scan gives not only topographic information but helps with "histologic differentiation." In addition, A scan can give hints concerning the compressibility and vascularity of the tumor. Although an exact histologic diagnosis cannot be made with A-scan ultrasound, this technique can usually distinguish between tumors, cysts, vascular anomalies, and inflammatory lesions.

B-scan ultrasound performed by the contact or water-bath method is more graphic in demonstrating the shape and size of lesions. Although easier to interpret spatially, it is less helpful with "histologic" differentiation. In most cases, therefore, the A scan emerges as the more complimentary adjunct to CT scanning. Since the technique and basic science of ultrasound are beyond the scope of this book, our discussion will be limited to specific examples of useful diagnostic characteristics and some pitfalls of ultrasonic examination.

Reflectivity

Internal reflectivity is a ratio between scattered, reflected, and transmitted energy. The physical characteristics of a tumor determine its reflectivity. Tissues containing compact cells with little intercellular structure (e.g., lymphoma) provide few reflective interfaces. The ultrasonic reflectivity will be low (Fig. 8-23). In contrast, tumors with large connective tissue interfaces, such as cavernous hemangiomas, will demonstrate high reflectivity (Fig. 8-24). Certain vascular malformations such as orbital varices and lymphargioma may exhibit alternating areas of high and low reflectivity (Fig. 8-25). The categories outlined in Table 8-1 will provide a rough guideline for the practitioner.

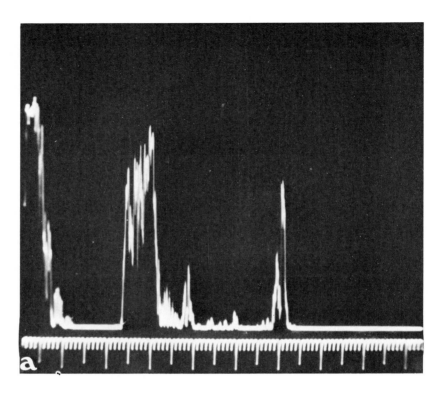

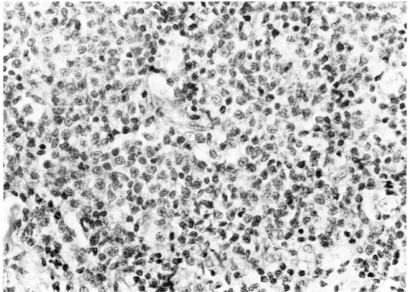

88

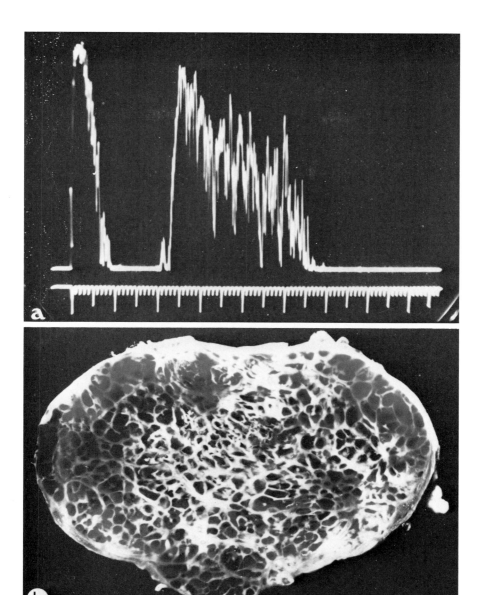

Fig. 8-24. (A) Medium to high reflectivity on A-scan ultrasonography. (B) Medium to high reflectivity is seen with tumors such as cavernous hemangioma. In this tumor, blood spaces are separated by connective tissue septa. The numerous tissue interfaces result in medium to high internal reflectivity.

Fig. 8-23. (A) A-scan ultrasonography showing lesion with low internal reflectivity. (B) Low internal reflectivity is seen with tumors such as malignant lymphoma, in which there are compact cells with little intercellular tissue structure.

89

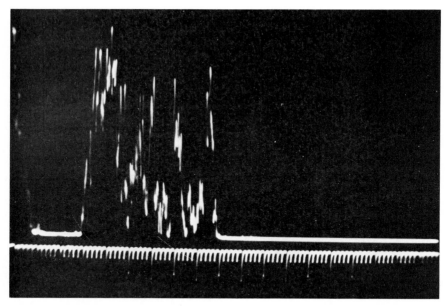

Fig. 8-25. A-scan ultrasonography with orbital lymphangioma. Cystic spaces within the tumor result in a pattern of alternating high and low internal reflectivity.

Table 8-1
Ultrasonic Reflectivity in Various Orbital Diseases

Low-reflectivity lesions

Lymphoma
Inflammatory pseudotumor
Dermoid cyst
Other cysts
Mucocele
Arteriovenous malformations
Chronic abscess
Chronic blood cyst

Medium-reflectivity lesions

Glioma
Meningioma
Subacute abscess
Subacute hemorrhage

High-reflectivity lesions

Cavernous hemangioma
Pleomorphic adenoma
Acute cellulitis or hemorrhage
Metastatic (area of low reflectivity centrally)

Table 8-1 (Continued)

Alternating high and low reflectivity

  Orbital varix
  Lymphangioma

Variable reflectivity

  Rhabdomyosarcoma
  Neurofibroma
  Neurilemmoma

Optic Nerve Changes

Thickness of the optic nerve and sheaths as determined on ultrasound (Fig. 8-26). can aid in the diagnosis of optic nerve tumors.

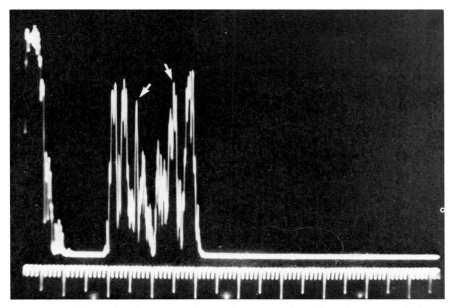

Fig. 8-26. Thickened optic nerve on A-scan ultrasonography with optic nerve meningioma.

Thickened Extraocular Muscles

The causes of increased extraocular muscle thickness include thyroid disease (common), inflammatory pseudotumor or myositis, arteriovenous fistulas, and metastatic disease (uncommon). One can measure muscle thickness with A scan (Fig. 8-27). Thickening of more than one muscle or one pair of muscles in the

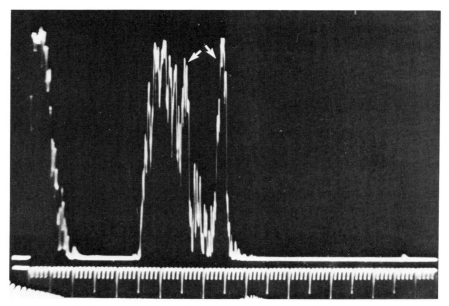

Fig. 8-27. Thickened lateral rectus muscle with A-scan ultrasonography.

appropriate clinical setting is highly suggestive of thyroid eye disease. In comparison, orbital myositis usually involves only one muscle.

Arteriovenous malformations produce secondary dilatation of the orbital veins. The veins in the extraocular muscles can dilate and again produce enlargement of more than one muscle on A scan. One must search for other clinical signs of fistulas, such as prominent episcleral vessels and an orbital bruit. In addition, enlargement of the superior ophthalmic vein may be detected. In such cases, fast, continuous echoes secondary to rapid blood flow may produce a "blurred" image on A scan. Other vascular tumors, such as hemangiopericytomas, can produce a similar "blurring" indicative of significant blood flow.

Metastatic disease involving just the extraocular muscles is uncommon. Standard tables outlining normal muscle width are available.*

Sinus Changes

Air represents a strong barrier to ultrasonic waves. Normal air-filled sinuses will deflect ultrasonic waves. Fluid collection or mucous membrane changes in a sinus will replace air and allow transmission of echo signals. Therefore,

*McNutt L: Ultrasound of Graves' Orbitopathy. Seminar, Department of Ophthalmology, University of Iowa, April 16, 1975

sinusitis, mucoceles, and sinus tumors can be detected with the A-scan method. Furthermore, the presence of defects in the anterior orbital walls can often be determined by ultrasonography.

Axial Length

A scan can be used to measure the axial length of the globe. Occasionally, axial myopia or arrested buphthalmos may produce the clinical picture of proptosis. This cause of pseudoproptosis can be ruled out rapidly with a modified A-scan technique.

Pitfalls of Ultrasound

Orbital ultrasound can detect foreign bodies, but localization in the orbit is difficult (Fig. 8-28). Other shortcomings of ultrasound include poor detection of orbital apex masses and inability to determine intracranial extension.

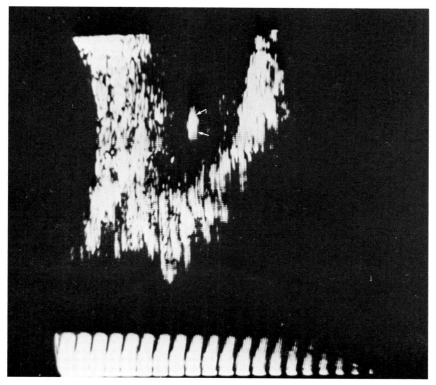

Fig. 8-28. B-scan ultrasonography shows wooden foreign body (arrows) in the center of an orbital abscess.

A double spike at the posterior edge of a lesion was previously thought to be highly characteristic of a cystic mass such as a dermoid cyst. This is only true if the double spike or "cyst wall" is seen in all meridians. A rapidly growing tumor such as a lymphoma can mimic a dermoid by displaying low reflectivity with a "pseudocyst wall" in one meridian (Fig. 8-29). The clinical history will often distinguish between these two lesions. Otherwise, it is crucial to examine the wall of the tumor in several meridians to rule out a "pseudocapsule" due to interaction of a rapidly growing tumor and normal orbital tissue.

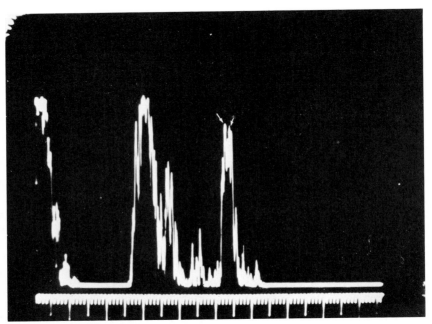

Fig. 8-29. "Double-spike" posterior wall typical of dermoid cyst (arrows). The double-spike wall was only seen in one meridian, however, and the patient had an orbital lymphoma. True orbital cysts should display double-spike posterior walls in more than one meridian of testing.

9
Surgery of the Orbit

Following investigation of the patient with orbital disease, a decision may be made to either observe the patient's condition or to institute medical therapy. Surgical management must also be considered. Surgical intervention in the orbit may be for (1) biopsy (incisional or excisional), a basically diagnostic procedure; (2) excision (partial or total), a therapeutic surgical maneuver; (3) drainage; (4) decompression; or (5) repair or reconstruction. The choice of the surgical manipulation will depend on the nature, location, extent, and activity of the disease process. Many excellent descriptions of surgical approaches to orbital diseases have been written. Much of the literature, however, has related the surgical approach to the histopathologic diagnosis. Unfortunately for the clinician, the histopathologic diagnosis usually awaits his or her surgical intervention and the obtaining of tissue. *Therefore, the ophthalmic surgeon must relate his or her surgical decision-making to the history, physical examination, and laboratory studies rather than to histopathologic diagnosis.* This requires generalized characterization of orbital lesions, to which can be added the various possibilities of surgical entry to the orbit (e.g., anterior orbitotomy, lateral orbitotomy). In this way a basic foundation for the surgical approach to diseases of the orbit can be established.

Useful characteristics for describing orbital lesions include location (anterior or posterior), extent (localized or diffuse), and biologic activity (nonprogressive or progressive). In assessing these characteristics, a careful physical examination and a review of laboratory studies are essential. The radiologist can tell us a great deal about the bony orbit based on plain x-rays, conventional tomography, and computerized tomographic (CT) scanning. CT scanning can relate the relationship of the abnormal lesion to the normal structures and anatomic planes of the orbit. Ultrasound also helps localize the lesion in addition to defining tissue types. These tests should be performed or reviewed by the orbital surgeon. One must not rely on a written report with a list of differential diagnostic possibilities. The orbital surgeon can best integrate the clinical and laboratory data by personally reviewing the test results with the radiologist or ultrasonographer.

NATURE OF ORBITAL LESIONS

Location

Orbital masses located in the anterior portion of the orbit are usually easily palpable and therefore readily accessible for biopsy or complete excision. These lesions frequently cause more globe displacement than actual proptosis. Their relationship to the bony orbit, orbital septum, and levator aponeurosis should be considered preoperatively, to guide the placement of the incision and technical approach to the lesion. Posterior orbital lesions are not readily accessible to palpation and generally cause more proptosis than displacement. Their relationship to the bony orbit, periorbita, muscle cone, and structures of the deep orbital apex including the optic foramen, should be delineated preoperatively. The equator of the globe might be considered an arbitrary anterior/posterior boundary defining the location of anterior and posterior intraorbital lesions.

Extent

The extent of orbital lesions is another important general characteristic. Localized lesions are more likely to be encapsulated, confined to a single surgical space, and totally resectable. Diffuse or infiltrative lesions will often cross multiple tissue planes and cause functional alterations of the eye and periocular tissue. They may not be amenable to total excision and are usually approached for incisional biopsy or orbital decompression.

Examples of lesions of histopathologic designation that may fit into the categories of location and extent include (1) anterior localized (dermoid cyst, benign mixed lacrimal gland tumor); (2) anterior diffuse (lymphoma, cellulitis); (3) posterior localized (cavernous hemangioma, optic nerve glioma); and (4) posterior diffuse (inflammatory pseudotumor, metastases).

Growth Parameters

The biologic activity or growth pattern of orbital lesions will also help the surgeon make decisions regarding timing and type of surgical intervention. Several parameters of biologic activity are: change in size, associated ocular dysfunction, and destruction of adjacent tissues. Progression of the size of a lesion may be demonstrated by changes in exophthalmometry readings and ocular displacement and by repeated CT or ultrasonic studies. Impairment of ocular function can be documented by a decrease in visual acuity, loss of visual field, abnormal pupillary response, change in color vision, change in refractive state, motility disturbance, or mass effect on the globe causing chorioretinal striae or scleral indentation. Destruction of surrounding tissues may cause radiographic abnormalities such as bony erosion, sinus opacification, or bony hyperostosis.

Lesions that are nonprogressive and have not had a significant effect on visual function can be observed. Lesions that are progressing, as documented by sequential examinations and laboratory studies, will be more amenable to definitive surgical treatment. The management of orbital lesions is determined not solely by presumed or confirmed histopathologic diagnosis but also by biologic activity. Even within a potential histopathologic diagnostic category, such as optic nerve glioma, decisions can be based on the activity of a particular lesion rather than on the classic description of its usual clinical behavior. This allows individualized treatment for each patient.

SURGICAL ENTRY TO THE ORBIT

Orbital surgery demands a thorough knowledge of orbital anatomy, including soft and bony tissues as well as eyelid anatomy. A working understanding of the surgical techniques involved in extensive eyelid, orbital soft-tissue, and bony manipulation is essential.

General anesthesia, with its present low risk of morbidity and mortality, is generally preferred. The exceptions are accessible anterior lesions, which can be approached with local infiltrative anesthesia. The use of controlled hypotension by the anesthesiologist in properly selected patients helps maintain a blood-free field and makes identification of vital structures and tissue planes easier. This is especially helpful in the orbital apex. The operating headlight, magnifying loupes, and operating microscope are essential for atraumatic dissection of intraorbital lesions. The technique of blunt finger dissection has been replaced by controlled, direct-vision dissection employing magnification, accessory intraorbital illumination, and meticulous hemostasis with a bipolar cautery unit.

Surgical entry to the orbit may be through the anterior or lateral approaches (Fig. 9-1).

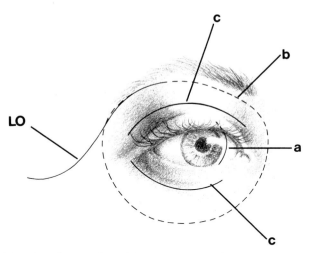

Fig. 9-1. Incision sites for anterior orbitotomy: transconjunctival approach—(a) "medial orbitotomy" (b) transcutaneous extraperiosteal approaches (c) transcutaneous trans-septal approaches and (LO) lateral orbitotomy.

Anterior Orbitotomy

Anterior orbitotomy may be done via the transcutaneous or transconjunctival approaches.

Transconjunctival Approach

The transconjunctival approach is useful for subconjunctival lesions and for lesions of the superior orbit deep to the levator aponeurosis. Lesions within or outside the muscle cone may be approached via this route. The rectus muscles may be disinserted from their insertions as necessary to allow entry to the muscle cone and visualization of the optic nerve.

The technical aspects of the transconjunctival approach are exemplified by the "medial" orbitotomy. The medial orbitotomy, often designated as a specific orbitotomy, is an anterior transconjunctival orbitotomy that involves a circumlimbal or radial conjunctival incision and disinsertion of the medial rectus muscle (transconjunctival approaches in other quadrants may involve disinsertion of other rectus muscles) (Fig. 9-2). This approach may be used for optic nerve biopsy, decompression, or complete excision of optic nerve tumors and other medial orbital lesions. A wire speculum, traction sutures, or Desmarres retractor is used to retract the eyelids. The eyelashes are not trimmed. Adhesive drapes may be used to exclude the lashes from the surgical field. Following the opening of the conjunctiva, sutures placed in the insertion of the medial rectus muscle, both on the globe and at the free end of the disinserted muscle, provide traction, which permits visualization of the intraconal space and optic

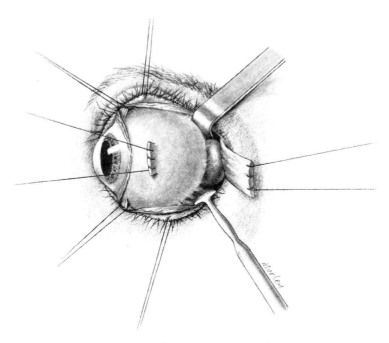

Fig. 9-2. Transconjunctival approach ("medial orbitotomy"); medial rectus muscle disinserted and retracted; globe abducted to facilitate exposure of retrobulbar structures. Note
intraconal tumor mass.

nerve. The superior and inferior rectus muscles may be looped with sutures to
aid in traction of the globe and improve exposure. Medial extraconal lesions will
not require the disinsertion of the rectus muscle. With gentle traction on these
sutures, dissection with appropriate illumination and magnification can be employed to displace orbital fat and visualize the lesion being approached. Careful
dissection can be undertaken before any cutting is done, using a fine, blunt-
tipped scissors with a spreading action. Tissue planes are spread to their thinnest
possible consistency to visualize vital structures (which can then be preserved)
or vascular channels (which can be cauterized prior to their transection).

The closure of the medial conjunctival approach includes reattachment of
the rectus muscle and closure of the conjunctiva by fine, buried, interrupted,
absorbable sutures. The conjunctival closure is not made watertight, to allow
seepage of blood and serum should they accumulate. The lids are closed prior
to the application of the dressing. Suture tarsorrhaphy is not performed. The
eyelids are covered by a Telfa pad. One oval eye pad is positioned and taped in
place. The Telfa pad is used to increase the ease of removing the dressing on the
first postoperative day. *No attempt at application of a pressure dressing is made.*
It is difficult, if not impossible, to apply a dressing that will truly tamponade

the orbital contents. Furthermore, attempts at placing this type of dressing may further compromise the vascular supply of the globe.

Patients are not routinely treated with systemic antibiotics. Systemic antibiotics are employed when an orbital infection is encountered or a sinus is exposed or drained. No specific postoperative limitations are imposed upon the patient other than those for routine periocular surgery. The dressing is removed on the first postoperative day, and the patient is discharged on the first or second postoperative day.

Transcutaneous Extraperiosteal Approach

The transcutaneous anterior orbitotomy may be done via the trans-septal or extraperiosteal routes.

The transcutaneous extraperiosteal anterior orbitotomy involves a skin incision positioned outside and parallel to the bony orbital rim (b, Fig. 9-1). The position and length of the skin incision depend on the site and size of the lesion. Generally, the incision is placed directly over the lesion. For superior orbital lesions the incision may be placed just beneath or in the inferior-most cilia of the eyebrow. Prior to making the skin incision, the proposed position is marked with a dye such as methylene blue or gentian violet. If local anesthesia is used, 1.5-percent lidocaine with 1:200,000 epinephrine is a good choice for local infiltration and/or specific nerve blocks. When general anesthesia is used, a small volume of 0.5-percent lidocaine with 1:200,000 epinephrine is often injected into the operative site to enhance hemostasis. The skin incision is carried through subcutaneous tissue and orbicularis oculi muscle, which is split in the direction of its fibers. Hemostasis is secured with the use of hemostats or with a cautery unit. Traction sutures of 4–0 silk are positioned in the superior and inferior aspects of the wound as necessary and attached to the drapes to provide traction and hemostasis. When the periosteum is encountered at the orbital rim, it is incised sharply and dissected off the bone with a periosteal elevator. The periosteal elevator modified by Tenzel, which has a Freer elevator at one end and a Cottle elevator at the other, is a useful instrument.

Once inside the bony margin, the extraperiosteal space (the potential space between periosteum and bone) is easily entered, and dissection is carried as posteriorly as necessary. Care must be exercised both laterally, to prevent injury to the lacrimal gland, and medially, to preserve the superior oblique muscle and trochlea. If necessary, the trochlea may be disinserted with the periosteum. Careful resuturing of the periosteum usually prevents motility disturbances. Laterally, one often encounters branches of the lacrimal artery and nerve, whereas medially the ethmoidal arteries are seen. The periosteum over a posterior lesion can then be incised. Palpation, biopsy, and/or decompression and drainage are accomplished as necessary. The periosteum (periorbita), however, must not be violated when dealing with extraperiosteal or sinus tumors, as this structure serves as a barrier protecting the soft-tissue orbital contents.

The wound (including periosteum at the orbital rim) is closed in layers. A soft rubber drain (such as a Penrose drain) is usually positioned, and placement is definitely indicated when blood or pus has been released or when extensive dissection has been done. Hemostasis should be meticulous. Visualization, particularly in deep orbital dissections, is enhanced by headlight illumination and magnifying loupes. Periosteal closure at the orbital margin is done with absorbable sutures such as catgut or polyglycolic acid (5-0). Muscle layers are reapproximated as necessary with similar sutures. In brow incisions particularly, the subcutaneous tissue may require several layers of interrupted buried sutures (e.g., 6-0 polyglycolic acid) to ensure that no tension is present on the cutaneous wound margins. The skin is closed with interrupted 6-0 or 7-0 fine silk sutures or running cutaneous or subcuticular sutures of 6-0 nylon or polypropylene. A light dressing is applied.

Systemic antibiotics are employed only when dealing with an orbital or sinus infection. Drains are advanced at the first dressing change and are usually discontinued on the morning of the second postoperative day. Visual acuity should be assessed at the first dressing change. The complaint of severe orbital pain in the early postoperative period must be evaluated immediately, since it may represent an orbital hemorrhage, which can be accompanied by visual loss. When orbital hemorrhage accompanied by visual loss occurs (orbital pain, proptosis, ecchymosis, reduced vision, Marcus-Gunn pupillary response), prompt orbital decompression must be accomplished. Accumulated blood is released by either opening the operative site or by more extensive decompressive procedures.

Transcutaneous Trans-septal Approach

The transcutaneous trans-septal anterior orbitotomy involves entering the orbit through the orbital septum (c, Fig. 9-1). This approach maintains the potential barrier of the periorbita. It is therefore indicated in those lesions suspected of being orbital malignancies. In this way, potential malignant spread into the extraperiosteal space is minimized. The skin incision is made over the preseptal orbicularis muscle within the confines of the orbital rims and above (or below) the tarsal border. Gentle traction placed on a suture in the lid margin may be used to facilitate the layered opening of the orbicularis muscle in the direction of the muscle fibers. Skin–muscle traction sutures are placed to improve exposure and hemostasis. Posterior digital pressure on the globe, which is protected with a methyl methacrylate corneal protector, will cause prolapse of orbital fat beneath the orbital septum. The septum can then be opened centrally with scissors placed tangentially to the bulging fat in a buttonhole fashion. A muscle hook may be placed beneath the orbital septum, applying upward traction; the orbital septum can then be opened across the horizontal extent of the lid with minimal risk to underlying structures. As the orbital septum is opened, care must be exercised not to damage the levator palpebrae superioris muscle or aponeurosis. After opening the orbital septum, intraorbital fat is encountered. Gentle palpation and blunt dissection of the orbital fat together with gentle pressure on the globe and careful placement of retractors will facilitate exposure. Carefully placed neurosurgical cottonoid strips are also useful in maintaining exposure.

After appropriate biopsy, excision, or drainage, the wound is closed in layers. The orbital septum is not closed as a separate layer, as it is reformed when the deep orbicularis muscle is reapproximated. A soft rubber drain is usually placed. Few, if any (buried, interrupted, absorbable) sutures are necessary to reapproximate the concentric fibers of the preseptal portion of the orbicularis muscle. The skin is closed with interrupted 6-0 or 7-0 silk sutures or with a running 6-0 polypropylene, nylon cutaneous, or subcuticular suture. A light dressing is applied, usually employing a Telfa pad and oval eye pad taped in place with 1-inch paper tape. Postoperative management is similar to that described for the extraperiosteal and transconjunctival anterior orbitotomies.

Orbital Endoscopy/Fine-Needle Aspiration

Orbital endoscopy and fine-needle aspiration biopsy are two other techniques of surgical entry to the orbit not involving removal of bone. Orbital endoscopy involves the use of an endoscope akin to an orthopedist's arthroscope. The endoscope has a total diameter of 1.7 mm including fiberoptic lighting and irrigation cannula. A system of instrumentation for use with the endoscope is available to facilitate observation of orbital structures and perform biopsy in selected cases. The endoscope can be helpful in removal of intraorbital foreign bodies and exploration of orbital tissue planes and lesions. This is accomplished with a small incision through skin or conjunctiva or in conjunction with other open surgical approaches.

Fine-needle aspiration biopsy involves the use of a 22- or 23-gauge needle attached to a syringe with a pistol-grip holder. This device allows the surgeon to apply strong aspiration pressure. Placement of the needle is achieved with ultrasonic or radiographic guidance. The aspiration biopsies performed with this technique require skilled cytologists to interpret the microscopic preparations. This technique is most valuable for diagnostic determinations of nonseeing eyes with optic nerve or suspected metastatic orbital tumors. Those disease processes such as lymphomatous lesions requiring careful pathologic review are not particularly amenable to cytologic diagnosis. Lacrimal gland tumors and tumors with a high fibrous tissue content do not lend themselves to fine-needle aspiration.

Fine-needle aspiration and orbital endoscopy are less invasive than open orbitotomy and may have increased application with improved instrumentation. At present, they must be considered a helpful addition to the orbital surgeon's armamentarium in a small number of selected cases.

Lateral Orbitotomy

The lateral orbitotomy is a transcutaneous orbitotomy involving temporary removal of a portion of the lateral orbital wall. This approach provides access to the retro-ocular spaces inside and outside the muscle cone for the surgical excision of orbital neoplasms and other lesions. In children it is preferable to avoid this procedure, to prevent bony growth disturbances. Fortunately, good surgical exposure without bone removal is usually possible in children, due to the more shallow configuration of the immature orbit. General endotracheal anesthesia is preferred. Induced intraoperative hypotension allows a bloodless field and is employed in patients in good physical condition.

The patient is positioned with the head slightly elevated and minimally rotated in the direction opposite the operative side. Sterile preparation is done in the region bounded by the hairline, nose, and upper lip. A traction suture can be positioned transconjunctivally in the lateral rectus muscle. The lids may be closed with a temporary traction suture, with suture tarsorrhaphy tied over cotton bolsters, or by sterile draping employing an adhesive plastic sheet. The site of skin incision is marked. The skin incision is curvilinear and extends from just beneath (or in) the inferior cilia of the lateral half of the eyebrow, which may be shaved without significant sequelae if desired. It is carried inferolaterally along the superior and lateral bony orbital rim past the level of the lateral commissure, ending over the zygomatic arch anterior to the hairline (Fig. 9-3a). Dissection is carried through the subcutaneous tissues and orbicularis oculi muscle to the level of the periosteum and fascia of the temporalis muscle. Hemostasis is initially controlled by pressure on the superior and inferior margins of the skin incision and with hemostats as necessary. The superior skin muscle flap is undermined, exposing the temporalis muscle fascia. The inferior flap is undermined, exposing the bony orbital rim. Traction sutures of 4–0 silk are positioned in the upper and lower flaps through the subcutaneous and muscularis tissue, avoiding unnecessary suture tracts through the skin. The traction sutures are secured to the drapes to effect exposure and aid in hemostasis. Hemostasis is further secured as necessary with cautery. The periosteum is then incised 2 mm behind and parallel to the lateral bony margin.

The incision is carried superiorly as far as the proposed bony excision (potentially as far as the supraorbital foramen) and inferiorly past the superior aspect of the zygomatic arch. The periosteal incision is then carried posteriorly along the zygomatic arch and along the upper part of the temporalis muscle, effecting its disinsertion by incising the periosteum superiorly and posteriorly (Fig. 9-3b). The periosteum is then stripped from the external aspect of the lateral orbital wall. The periosteum and temporalis muscle are reflected posteriorly from the zygomatic process of the frontal bone and the frontal process of the zygomatic bone. This exposes the fossa of the temporalis muscle and the bone of the lateral orbital wall. The joining of superior and inferior periosteal

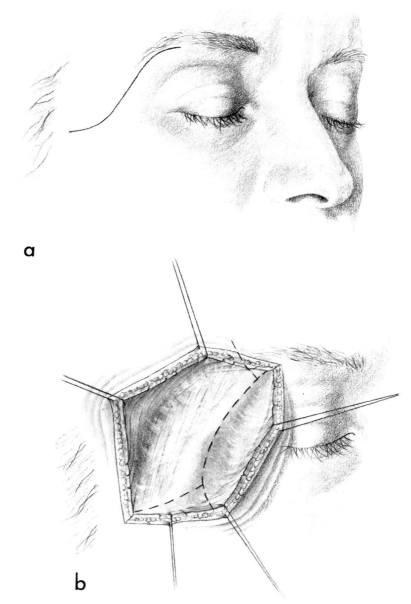

a

b

Fig. 9-3.   Lateral orbitotomy. (a) Skin incision. (b) Retraction of skin-muscle with traction sutures. Periosteal incision with superior and inferior relaxing incisions. (c) Reflection of periosteum and temporalis muscle. (d) Drill holes placed on both sides of the intended upper and lower edges of proposed bony incision.

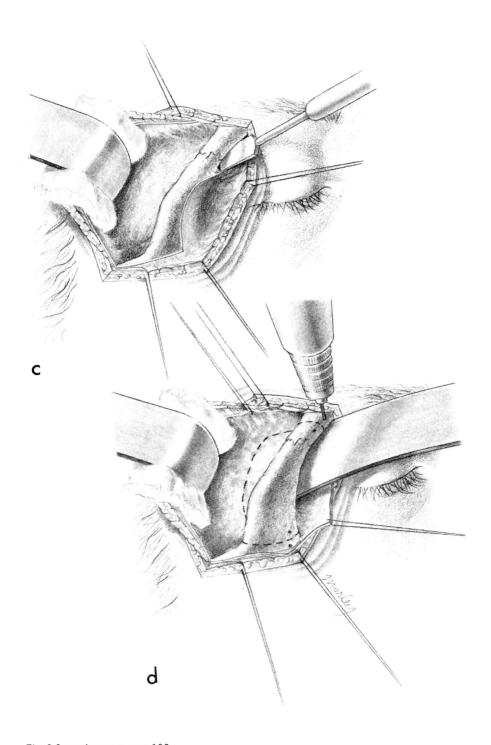

c

d

Fig. 9-3 continues on page 108.

incisions to the marginal periosteal incision allows this posterior displacement of the temporalis muscle. The blunt dissection of the temporalis muscle requires firm pressure and further relaxation of the periosteal incisions. Disinsertion of the muscle superiorly may be necessary. Brisk venous bleeding may be encountered in the bed of the temporalis muscle. This can ususally be controlled by pressure. Dissection of the periosteum and subsequently the excision of bone is carried superiorly (and posteriorly) as far as necessary for the indications of the procedure (Fig. 9-3c). An extensive resection of a tumor of the fossa of the lacrimal gland would require greater bony excision ("extended" lateral orbitotomy) than necessary for the resection of a localized intraconal cavernous hemangioma. Knowledge of the location of the frontal sinuses is mandatory. The periorbita is then freed from the inner orbital wall. The periorbita is loosely applied to the inner wall and can be easily separated from bone as far posteriorly as the orbital apex.

A broad malleable retractor is then positioned in the orbit along the lateral wall. This protects the orbital soft tissue contents while drill holes are made with a pneumatic drill on either side of the intended upper and lower edges of the bony incisions (Fig. 9-3d). The bone incisions can then be made with an oscillating saw. The lower cut is placed along the upper margin of the zygomatic arch. The upper cut is positioned above the frontozygomatic suture. A third cut is placed in the fossa of the temporalis muscle joining the superior and inferior rim cuts (Fig. 9-3e). During the bone-cutting, malleable retractors over gauze pads or wide neurosurgical cottonoid patties are used to retract the temporalis muscle and associated soft tissue. Irrigating fluid is used to prevent heat necrosis of the bone. Suction is employed to prevent widespread scattering of bony fragments. The saw cuts are positioned slightly more superior on the outer aspect of the bony wall to allow a snug template-like fit when the bone fragment is replaced. The lateral wall fragment is then grasped at the rim with a large clamp and gently rocked and elevated. The bony fragment is fractured and removed from its site (Fig. 9-3f). It is placed in warm lactated Ringer's solution and saved for later replacement. Further bony resection may be accomplished in the depths of the fossa of the temporalis muscle using rongeurs or a pneumatic drill with diamond burr. Bone wax may be used to control bleeding. The bony opening can be enlarged posteriorly, superiorly, and inferiorly back to the thick bone protecting the middle cranial fossa. This technique is particularly useful for improving visualization with superior and apical orbital lesions ("extended" lateral orbitotomy).

Further retraction of the temporalis muscle may be accomplished at this point with traction sutures or retractors. The intact periorbita can then be visualized. The periorbita is incised anterioposteriorly below the level of the inferior aspect of the lacrimal gland and approximately at the level of the upper border of the lateral rectus muscle. A vertical incision in the periorbita anteriorly is also made, effecting a "T"-shaped periorbita incision. Relaxing incisions in the posteriormost aspect of the periorbita may also be made as necessary in a

"Y" or "T" shape. The orbit can then be carefully palpated and the position of any mass determined. The lateral rectus muscle may be identified by direct visualization and opening of the perimuscular fascial sheaths. When identified, the lateral rectus muscle may be looped with a traction suture of umbilical tape or surgical silicone bands (Fig. 9-3g).

Intraorbital dissection can then be performed with an operating microscope or operating loupes and the fiberoptic headlight. Intraorbital structures should be identified by careful dissection and divided only under direct visualization with application of cautery when necessary. Hemostasis must be meticulous. Following removal of intraorbital tumors or the performance of necessary intraorbital procecures, closure begins with the placement of absorbable sutures in the anterior aspect of the periorbita. Chromic catgut (4-0 or 5-0) or polyglycolic acid (5-0 or 6-0) is useful for this closure. No attempt is made to provide a watertight closure. Proper drainage of accumulated blood or other tissue fluids must be allowed. The lateral orbital wall bone fragment is replaced and fixed in position with 3-0 stainless steel wire (Fig. 9-3h). The wire is placed in the previously drilled holes and twisted to proper tightness to ensure a satisfactory alignment. The ends of the wire are cut long enough to allow them to be bent into the drill holes on the external surface of the bony rim. The bone fragment may not fit tightly in place if the posterior bony opening was widened with the rongeur or burr. A soft rubber drain (such as the Penrose drain) or a suction drainage system is positioned in the fossa of the temporalis muscle. This drain is brought out inferior to the lateral aspect of the incision through a separate stab wound.

The temporalis muscle is returned to its position in the temporalis fossa, and the periosteum and anterior temporalis fascia are reapproximated with buried interrupted sutures of 3-0 or 4-0 chromic catgut or 5-0 polyglycolic acid (Fig. 9-3i). Traction sutures are removed. Muscle and subcutaneous tissues are then reapproximated with multiple interrupted sutures of 5-0 or 6-0 polyglycolic acid. A running subcuticular or cutaneous suture of 6-0 nylon or 6-0 polypropylene is then used to close the skin incision. (This may be augmented by several widely spaced interrupted sutures.) The drain is secured to the skin with an interrupted suture (Fig. 9-3j). Traction sutures in the tendon of the lateral rectus muscle or temporary tarsorrhaphy sutures are removed. The incision is dressed with a folded 4 by 4 gauze over a Telfa pad. The eye may be patched with an oval eye pad. No attempt is made to apply a "pressure" dressing. A head-wrap type dressing is not applied. The drain site is similarly dressed. A short course of systemic antibiotics is given. The dressing is removed in 24 hours. The drain is advanced and removed in 24 to 48 hours. Skin or subcuticular sutures are removed in 5 to 10 days. When skin sutures are removed early, steri-strips are placed to aid wound closure and stability.

The postoperative period may be characterized by periorbital edema, ecchymosis, ptosis, extraocular muscle imbalance, and hypesthesia. These findings can be expected to resolve with minimal residua. Complications may include

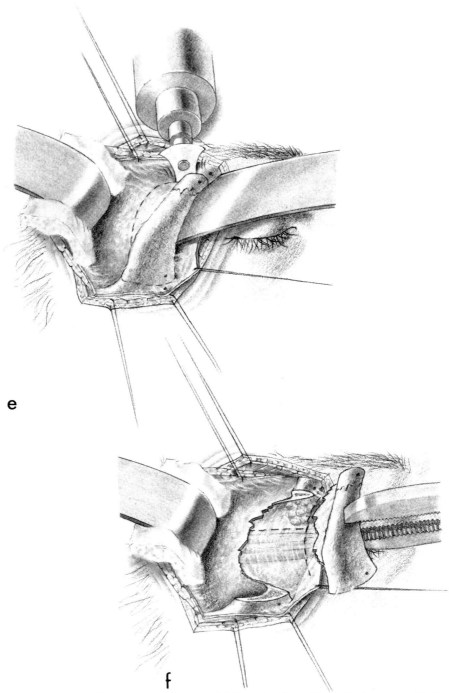

Fig. 9-3 (continued). Lateral orbitotomy. (e) Bone incision with oscillating saw; orbital structures protected with malleable ribbon retractor. (f) Removal of lateral bony orbital wall fragment. Note proposed incision site on periorbita and its relationship to the lateral rectus

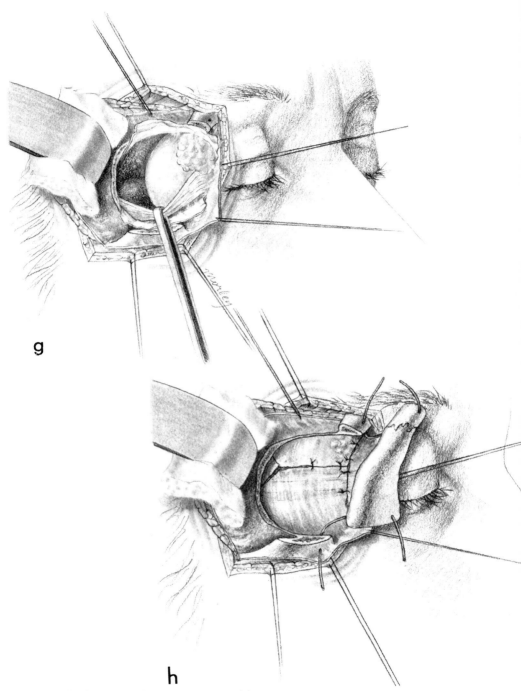

g

h

muscle and orbital lobe of the lacrimal gland. (g) Bony incision enlarged, periorbita incised, lateral rectus identified and retracted allowing access to intraconal space. (h) Periorbita closed and bone fragment replaced and fixated with stainless steel wires.

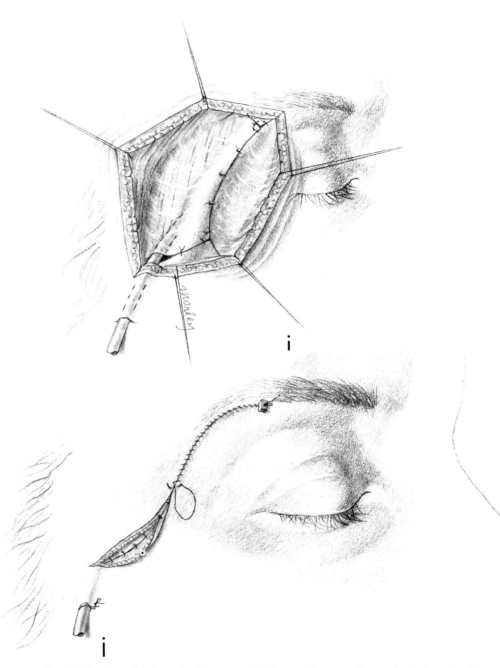

Fig. 9-3 (continued). Lateral orbitotomy. (i) Closure of temporalis muscle fascia and periosteum with drain in place. (j) Layered soft tissue closure. Drain brought out through separate incision and secured to skin.

hemorrhage, inflammation, infection, optic atrophy, cranial nerve injury, extraocular muscle imbalance, ptosis, and/or injury to the lacrimal gland, perinasal sinuses, cranial vault, or the eye itself.

Proper orbital drainage will reduce the risk of an extensive intraorbital accumulation of blood or tissue fluid. Gentle traction on extraocular muscles will minimize the risk of motility disturbances. The systemic use of steroids when inflammatory lesions are encountered or when a dermoid cyst ruptures will shorten the period of postoperative swelling and reaction. Traction or pressure on the optic nerve or posterior ocular blood supply should be limited to very short intervals (less than 2 minutes) to reduce the possibility of visual loss. Self-retaining retractors, if used, must be frequently released and repositioned to prevent optic nerve ischemia.

Visual loss secondary to persistent intraorbital postoperative hemorrhage must be managed aggressively. Ultrasonographic evaluation may demonstrate a loculated area of hemorrhage. When identified in the presence of visual loss, localized accumulations should be drained immediately. This can be done by opening the initial incision or through another approach. Intraconal decompression via a transconjunctival medial orbitotomy should be considered in the presence of visual loss and afferent pupillary defect when no extraconal or loculated hemorrhage is identified.

Complications of orbital surgery can in part be limited by meticulous surgical technique; however, complications cannot be totally avoided. Further problems such as intraocular hemorrhage, retinal detachment, optic atrophy, pupillary abnormalities, sinus fistula, and cerebrospinal fluid leak are fortunately uncommon.

Exenteration

Orbital exenteration is indicated for malignant neoplasms that are confined to the orbit and not totally responsive to chemotherapy and/or radiotherapy. Orbital exenteration involves the surgical removal of the entire orbital contents, including the periorbita and all tissue confined within the periorbita. Following this removal, the remnants of deep apical orbital structures as well as the nasolacrimal duct are extensively cauterized. The palpebral conjunctiva and eyelid structures may be preserved when not involved by deep orbital tumors. Malignant lacrimal gland tumors with apparent involvement of the bone on x-ray require extensive removal of orbital bone to the level of dura. This type of surgery should be done in cooperation with neurosurgeons and plastic surgeons. Following exenteration with bone excision, reconstruction usually involves the rotation of a local (scalp) flap or a distant (arm) flap to cover exposed dura and fill the orbital cavity. When the bone remains intact, the orbital cavity may be covered with a skin graft or filled partially with a temporalis muscle flap and thereafter covered with a skin graft. Our preferred technique involves healing by primary epithelialization and granulation of the socket. This technique eliminates the need of obtaining skin graft material or repositioning flaps and avoids the problem of desquamating skin in the orbital cavity following skin graft healing. The initial several weeks to months following surgery may require greater attention in the granulating socket than in the skin grafted socket. The long-term advantages, however, of the socket epithelialized by primary intention with nonkeratinizing epithelium are significant, in our judgment.

In all circumstances, decisions to perform radical extirpative surgery should be based on the study of permanently fixed histopathologic specimens, not on frozen section tissue study. The major value of frozen sections in the surgical management of orbital disease is in indicating to the surgeon whether obtained tissue is representative of a tumor mass. This may be helpful in instances in which orbital fat may be confused with tumor, such as in cases of lymphoma or inflammatory psuedotumor. Frozen sections may also be used, as is commonly done in the surgery of basal cell carcinoma of the eyelids, to define adequate margins of resection.

SELECTION OF SURGICAL APPROACH
TO ORBITAL LESIONS

Given the generalized nature of orbital lesions confronting the ophthalmic surgeon and the various possible approaches to entering the orbit, a framework of decision-making can be proposed. A summary of surgical options is represented in Table 9-1. This chart is not all-inclusive, but hopefully it will help provide a rational approach to a complex problem.

Anterior lesions, both localized and diffuse, may be approached surgically via anterior (including medial) orbitotomies. Localized anterior lesions can usually undergo an excisional biopsy (total excision). Total excision of a lesion should be done when it is technically possible. Diffuse infiltrative lesions in the anterior orbit should undergo incisional biopsy. Biopsy provides a definitive diagnosis before therapy and may suggest the primary site of a secondary or metastatic lesion. Infectious lesions in the anterior orbit are amenable to drainage and decompression, as are localized blood cysts.

Lesions in the posterior orbit may also be approached for incisional biopsy, total excision, drainage, or decompression via anterior or lateral orbitotomy. When total excision is unnecessary or impossible, as with diffuse lesions such as extensive orbital varices, inflammatory pseudotumor, metastatic lesions, or suspected infiltrative malignancies, surgery should be designed to remove only that tissue necessary for diagnosis or decompression. This may be accomplished through the anterior approach or possibly via endoscopy or fine-needle aspiration. Localized progressive lesions evidenced by increasing proptosis and/or decreasing visual function that are not suspected of being inflammatory should be explored via the anterior or lateral route, as indicated. Medial lesions or optic

Table 9-1
Selection of Surgical Approach for Orbital Lesions

Approach	Nature of Lesion	Examples	Possible Operations
Anterior orbitotomy	Anterior, localized	Dermoid cyst	Excision
	Anterior, diffuse	Lymphoma, anterior orbital abscess	Biopsy, drainage
	Posterior, diffuse	pseudotumor, posterior orbital abscess, metastatic lesion, lymphoma	Biopsy, drainage
	Lacrimal gland lesions (not clinically benign mixed)	Malignant carcinoma of lacrimal gland	Biopsy
Medial orbitotomy	Medial, anterior, localized	Vascular abnormality (varix, hemangioma)	Excision, biopsy
	Medial, posterior, localized	Cavernous hemangioma, pseudotumor	Excision, biopsy
	Medial, anterior, diffuse	Orbital abscess, rhabdomyosarcoma	Drainage, biopsy
	Optic nerve lesion	Optic nerve glioma, meningioma	Biopsy, excision, decompression
Endoscopy	Localized, posterior	Orbital foreign body	Removal
	Diffuse, posterior	Pseudotumor, metastatic lesion	Biopsy
	Optic nerve lesion	Glioma, meningioma	Biopsy
Fine-needle aspiration biopsy	Diffuse, posterior	Malignant sarcoma	Biopsy
	Optic nerve lesion	Glioma, meningioma	Biopsy
Lateral orbitotomy	Posterior, localized (intraconal or extraconal)	Meningioma, hemangioma	Biopsy, excision
	Posterior, diffuse	Metastatic lesion, pseudotumor	Biopsy, decompression, drainage
"Extended" lateral orbitotomy	Localized, posterior, apical	Meningioma	Excision, biopsy
	Lacrimal gland fossa lesions	Benign mixed lacrimal gland tumor	Excision with adjacent tissue
Exenteration	Extensive, malignant, orbital lesions	Lacrimal gland carcinoma, sarcomatous lesions	Excision with orbital contents

113

nerve lesions may be reached via a medial transconjunctival orbitotomy. Lateral orbitotomy is usually required for the total excision of posterior tumor masses. Nonprogressive lesions of the posterior orbit not associated with visual loss may be observed for evidence of activity and progression. An extended lateral orbitomy is useful when dealing with tumors in the orbital apex.

SURGICAL PEARLS

The following points should be considered by the orbital surgeon:

1. The standard retinal or lens cryoprobe can be extremely useful in orbital surgery. It enables the surgeon to exert traction on a tumor while minimizing the chance of inadvertently rupturing a tumor capsule. However, the probe does not substitute for meticulous blunt dissection along tissue planes within the orbit.
2. Although it is generally preferred to excise a tumor completely with the capsule intact, one can place traction sutures *into* a cavernous hemangioma to aid in removal. The sutures provide traction and allow escape of blood. This maneuver shrinks the size of the mass, facilitating removal. Bleeding from the tumor will usually stop in several minutes. In order to perform this maneuver, one must be familiar with the clinical, radiographic, ultransonic, and operative characteristics of the cavernous hemangioma. This procedure should not be performed when a malignant lesion is suspected.
3. It is usually impossible to totally resect diffusely infiltrative lesions such as capillary hemangiomas, orbital varices, or plexiform neurofibromas without damaging vital structures. A limited "debulking" of such tumors usually affords a satisfactory cosmetic appearance with preservation of function.
4. Rupturing the capsule of a dermoid cyst can lead to a marked inflammatory response that may become chronic. Dermoid tumors will frequently extend quite posteriorly, especially in adults. The surgeon must always be prepared to extend the original incision or undertake a large orbitotomy when dealing with these cysts. This includes cases in which a palpable mass is encountered and the tumor is seemingly limited to the anterior compartment. These tumors can extend into the intracranial space, making neurosurgical assistance mandatory.
5. Subconjunctival lipodermoids of the superior temporal quadrant may extend posteriorly. Excision is occasionally undertaken for cosmetic reasons. Dissection should be limited to that portion of the lesion that is clinically visible through the open palpebral aperture. This will minimize the risk of injury to deep orbital structures such as levator aponeurosis, lacrimal gland, and extraocular muscles. The risk of globe perforation and symblepharon formation is also minimized.

6. Closure of an orbitotomy should not commence until complete hemostasis has been accomplished. In some instances this may require not only careful cauterization of visible bleeding points but also the use of topical clotting agents. The orbital surgeon should be familiar with these agents.
7. Bipolar cautery is preferred in orbital surgery. It enables one to work in a wet field and reduces the risk of current being transmitted to adjacent normal tissue.
8. It is usually not necessary to type and crossmatch blood in preparation for orbital surgery. Notable exceptions include patients with blood dyscrasias and those who are anticoagulated. Inhibitors of platelet aggregation, including aspirin, should be stopped one week before surgery.

10
Management of Common Orbital Diseases

THYROID OPHTHALMOPATHY

Thyroid ophthalmopathy can pose a frustrating problem for both patient and physician because of the chronicity and vacillating nature of the disorder. The ophthalmologic symptoms of the vast majority of these patients stabilize or resolve spontaneously in several months, although the symptoms may wax and wane for several years. The importance of close interaction between orbital consultant and endocrinologist cannot be overemphasized. It is generally agreed that correction of any systemic thyroid hormone imbalance is necessary if clinical stability is to be attained.

The hallmarks of thyroid ophthalmopathy are proptosis, lid lag with lid retraction, chemosis, and injection (often limited to the lateral rectus muscle). Motility disturbances are common and usually manifest as impaired elevation or abduction of the eye. *Thyroid ophthalmopathy is the most common cause of both unilateral and bilateral proptosis.* This disease is encountered mainly in adulthood. The spectrum of disease is broad, with findings varying from mild palpebral edema to visual loss secondary to optic neuropathy. Onset of symptoms may be insidious or fulminate.

Medical Treatment

The frequently reported symptoms of foreign-body sensation result from exposure and dryness caused by proptosis, lid retraction, and decreased blinking. These symptoms are treated with topical lubricants. The use of drops during waking hours and liberal application of ointment at bedtime will minimize

117

corneal irritation. Palpebral or conjunctival edema may be lessened by elevating the head during sleep with pillows or bed blocks.

Severe, acute corneal exposure may be temporarily treated with a moisture chamber. Plastic wrap (e.g., Saran wrap) or a similar material may be used to create a form-fitting, inexpensive moisture chamber. Vaseline or tape is used to seal the contact of plastic wrap to skin around the orbital margins.

Systemic steroids play a definite role in the management of the more severe problems, such as optic neuropathy and corneal exposure with exophthalmos. Steroids should be tried as the initial form of therapy in cases where the integrity of the cornea and/or optic nerve is threatened. Steroid doses may range from 40 to 120 mg/day of prednisone. Results are usually evident within 24 to 48 hours in responsive patients. The dose may then be tapered to every-other-day therapy and titrated as the clinical situation dictates. The high doses should not be maintained for longer than 7 to 10 days in nonresponsive patients. If no response to steroids is apparent, irradiation and/or surgery should be considered. Treatment over weeks to months with a reduced dosage may be necessary to control symptoms in steroid-responsive patients.

A solution of 5- to 10-percent guanethidine has sympatholytic properties, which would seem to render it useful for the treatment of lid retraction. However, its efficacy after administration is short-lived. Furthermore, the side effects of miosis, myopia, and punctuate keratitis make patient compliance difficult. Thymoxamine, an alpha-adrenergic blocking agent, may prove useful in the medical treatment of eyelid retraction.

Surgical Treatment

The indications for surgery in patients with thyroid ophthalmopathy include severe eyelid retraction with exposure keratopathy, diplopia with extraocular muscle restrictions, "malignant" congestive exophthalmos, and optic neuropathy unresponsive to systemic steroids and orbital irradiation.

Muscle Surgery

Clinically the inferior rectus muscle is most commonly affected. Fibrosis secondary to inflammatory changes may contract the muscle, causing hypotropia, limitation of upgaze, and accentuation of upper lid retraction. Symptoms and signs should be stable for at least 6 to 12 months prior to surgery to increase the possibility that a satisfactory result will not be transient because of continued disease activity. Recession of the inferior rectus muscle with adjustable sutures may be useful in selected patients. Lower eyelid retraction may follow large inferior rectus recessions if the attachments between inferior rectus and lower lid are not released. Medial rectus restriction is the second most common motility problem seen. Superior rectus restriction is occasionally encountered. Prisms may be used postoperatively to correct small residual deviations.

Eyelid Surgery

Upper eyelid retraction may be caused by sympathetic overinnervation of the upper lid retractors (Fig. 10-1). Surgical alternatives include levator recession with or without scleral graft interposition. The latter procedure consists of interposition of fresh or preserved eye bank sclera between the tarsus and recessed eyelid retractors. Scleral graft interposition may also be used for correction of lower eyelid retraction. Medial and lateral taronhaphies and canthoplasties may also be useful.

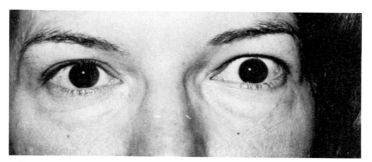

Fig. 10-1.   Lid retraction on the left side with thyroid ophthalmopathy.

Orbital Decompression

Surgical decompression of the orbit may be required when either the cornea or optic nerve is acutely threatened. Orbital decompression for cosmetic reasons is occasionally done, but it involves significant risks. The major complications are diplopia and paresthesias in the distribution of the infraorbital nerve. The surgeon must balance the risk of complications with the cosmetic indication. If surgery is elected, decompression may be done by removal of the lateral, inferior, and medial orbital walls. Concomitant opening of the periorbita allows release of intraorbital contents. The amount of surgery must be tailored to the specific patient. The transcranial approach is not recommended. Those procedures disrupting the orbital floor and medial wall via a transconjunctival, transcutaneous, or transantral (Caldwell-luc) approach are preferred.

Radiation Therapy

The use of radiation therapy must also be considered in management of certain patients (Table 10-1). X-ray therapy has provided an alternative to long-term steroid use. Irradiation may prevent a clinical relapse when steroid dosages are tapered. Those patients unresponsive to a short, intensive course of systemic steroids (two to three weeks or less in severe cases) should be treated with either orbital irradiation or surgical decompression. Effects of irradiation (1500 to

Table 10-1
Management of Thyroid Eye Disease

	Findings				
				Exposure Keratopathy	
	Ocular Irritation	Diplopia With EOM Restriction	Lid Retraction and Exophthalmos	Mild to Moderate / Moderate to Severe	Optic Neuropathy
Treatment	Topical lubricants; Moisture chamber	Prisms	Eyelid retractor recession; lateral and/or medial tarsorrhaphy, canthoplasty	Topical lubricants, moisture chamber (Mild to Moderate); Systemic corticosteroids (Moderate to Severe)	Systemic corticosteroids
		Extraocular muscle surgery		Orbital decompression eyelid surgery	Orbital decompression
				Irradiation	Irradiation

120

2000 rads) are usually evident in several weeks, although some patients respond in three to five days. Supervoltage irradiation may be effectively delivered by a well collimated Cobalt-60 unit or a linear accelerator.

Treatment of thyroid ophthalmopathy is summarized in Table 10-1.

CAPILLARY HEMANGIOMA

The most frequent vascular tumors or malformations are capillary hemangioma, orbital varix, lymphangioma, cavernous hemangioma, and orbital blood cyst secondary to orbital hemorrhage.

Capillary hemangiomas often present within the first few weeks of life, with approximately one third present at birth. Significant growth can occur over several months. Characteristically, the lesion is dark-red or bluish in color, rather spongy in consistency, and diffuse (Fig. 10-2). Hemangiomas may be noted on the forehead, trunk, or palate. Plain skull x-rays will often reveal a diffusely enlarged orbit. Orbital ultrasonography may confirm the diagnosis of vascular lesion. However, the diagnosis is often based on clinical criteria alone. The CT scan can be helpful in delineating the size of the lesion but is not usually necessary for diagnosis.

The capillary hemangioma may be an especially challenging management problem. The usual course of this lesion is spontaneous resolution. Approximately 75 percent resolve by 7 years of age; therefore, most of these lesions can best be managed by attentive neglect. The indications for therapeutic or diagnostic intercession include (1) a high index of suspicion of another tumor (most frequently rhabdomyosarcoma), (2) amblyopia secondary to anisometropia

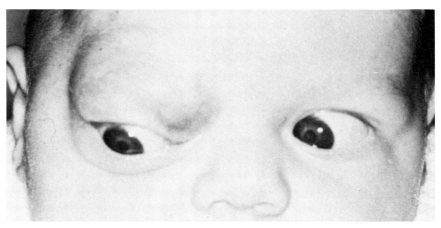

Fig. 10-2. Diffuse involvement of the right upper eyelid with a capillary hemangioma. The right globe is displaced downward.

(induced cylinder caused by tumor compression), strabismus, or (rarely) marked blepharoptosis, and (3) cosmetic improvement. Amblyopia is the most frequent complication of capillary hemangioma. The use of spectacles to correct induced astigmatism and patching of the noninvolved eye may be a necessary adjunct to medical or surgical therapy. The cosmetic blemish of a capillary hemangioma in an infant can be extremely stressful to the parents. This does not usually constitute an indication for intervention because of the trend towards spontaneous resolution and the possible complications of both medical and surgical therapy.

Treatment modalities used have included surgical excision, corticosteroid therapy, radiotherapy, sclerosing agents, radon implants, direct application of solid carbon dioxide, and ligation of afferent vessels. The most useful modalities are corticosteroid therapy, surgery, and low-dose radiotherapy.

Systemic steroids should be the initial form of therapy for large diffuse masses. Steroid therapy must be given in cooperation with a pediatrician. Exacerbation may occur even when steroids are slowly tapered. Clinical response should be evident within a week. Steroids should not be continued beyond ten days to two weeks if no response is seen. Results of steroid treatment are variable. The improvement seen in many patients is transient. Limited surgical debulking can be done when steroid treatment has been unsuccessful. No attempt at total excision of these large, diffuse lesions should be attempted. Surgery is also indicated for persistent, well-demarcated, nondiffuse tumors and for those causing a diagnostic dilemma.

Radiotherapy with superficial orthovoltage techniques, in doses of 100 to 500 rads, has been useful in reducing tumor mass. Side effects may be minimized with appropriate shielding of the globe. Possible complications ranging from cataract to periorbital skin changes may occur.

Treatment can do more harm than good and should be initiated only when necessary. The use of implanted radioactive sources, injection of sclerosing agents, or the use of high-dose irradiation should be avoided. Localized periocular steroid injections and photocoagulation have also been used in the management of capillary hemangiomas. These modalities deserve careful study as to their efficacy.

VARIX AND LYMPHANGIOMA

The orbital varix and lymphangioma can be considered together, since clinical presentation and management of these lesions are similar and pathologic differentiation is often difficult. These lesions may present in one of four ways: (1) enlarged veins in the lids or conjunctiva but no proptosis, (2) variable proptosis with no visible lesions, (3) variable proptosis with dilated veins in the lids and episcleral tissues, and (4) acute orbital hemorrhage (Fig. 10-3).

The best management approach for patients in the first three groups is

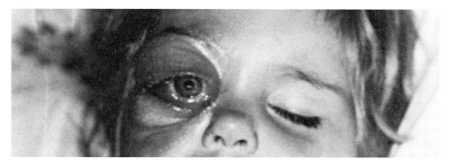

Fig. 10-3. Acute orbital hemorrhage on the right side in a patient with an orbital varix.

simple observation. Indications for surgery in this group are primarily cosmetic, but also include eyelid malposition or visual disturbances from an induced astigmatism. Excision of dilated veins in the lids and conjunctiva may be sufficient. The venous abnormalities should be isolated with meticulous dissection. Hemostasis is obtained with ligature and cautery as necessary.

Indication for excision of posterior orbital varices is limited to patients with recurrent, painful episodes of orbital hemorrhage. Excision of deep orbital varices for cosmesis is avoided because of the high incidence of visual loss and damage to deep orbital structures. Patients with recurrent orbital hemorrhage and repeated venous thromboses of the orbit may develop the "orbital strangulation" syndrome with visual loss and chronic pain. Unlike the responsive capillary hemangioma, steroids and radiation therapy play no role in the management of patients with varices and lymphangiomas.

The management of the patient with acute hemorrhage begins with attention to vision and corneal exposure. Visual acuity must be obtained. The pupillary responses and optic discs should be carefully evaluated. Investigation of bleeding disorder parameters should be pursued. The optic nerve and central retinal artery are usually not irreversibly compromised, especially in children, since the venous bleeds are self-tamponaded at pressures below arterial levels. Most patients can be managed conservatively with close observation. Temporary tarsorrhaphy utilizing steri-strips at the lid margins can be useful when there is significant corneal exposure in the absence of optic nerve compression. The steri-strips are built up as pyramids with bases at the upper and lower lid margins. Silk sutures (4-0) are then placed through the bases of the triangles and tied, creating a tarsorrhaphy.

The presence of an afferent pupillary defect or documented visual loss demands immediate surgical intervention. Adequate decompression must be accomplished and maintained for 24 to 48 hours following surgery. Needle drainage is not advocated, for it will usually only provide temporary relief. Orbital ultrasound (and in some cases, venography) may be used to help define a localized accumulation of blood. A transconjunctival or transcutaneous approach may be used depending on the extent and suspected location of the hemorrhage. The surgeon must be prepared to decompress the extraconal and intraconal space. A soft rubber drain or gentle suction drainage may be employed following exploration.

Management of the elderly patient with spontaneous orbital hemorrhage is often complicated by a secondary vascular occlusion or arterial bleed. The time sequence from occurrence of hemorrhage to irreversible visual loss in the elderly is usually too short to allow effective therapy. However, if the patient is seen within hours of a hemorrhage with documented visual loss, immediate surgical drainage is recommended. Further measures such as paracentesis may be indicated when there is a secondary central retinal artery occlusion.

The patient presenting with a suspected blood cyst that is slowly enlarging must be surgically explored to rule out an orbital neoplasm. Ultrasonography and computerized tomography will accurately localize the lesion and dictate the surgical approach. A transconjunctival or transcutaneous approach may be used. Adequate drainage must be maintained for at least 24 hours after removel of the walls and contents of the blood cyst. Proper evacuation and drainage will reduce the incidence of visual loss from potential rebleeding.

CAVERNOUS HEMANGIOMA

The encapsulated, well-circumscribed, cavernous hemangioma is the most common primary orbital tumor in adults. This tumor usually presents in early middle-age. The most frequent presenting sign is gradually increasing, nonvariable, painless proptosis followed by a decrease of visual acuity often interpreted by the patient as a distortion of vision. The course of the disease process is measured in years. There is usually no chemosis or injection, and proptosis is usually axial. Ophthalmoscopy may reveal choroidal folds and variable optic nerve changes including mild swelling, blurring of the disc margins, and temporal pallor. Skull x-rays are usually normal. Ultrasonography and CT scanning can confirm the vascular nature and location of the mass.

While this intraconal tumor is histopathologically benign, surgery should not be deferred for a long period of time when signs of progression are present. A lateral orbitotomy is usually indicated for complete excision of this intraconal tumor.

Large arterial feeder vessels are rarely encountered at surgery, as cavernous hemangiomas represent hamartomas of venous origin. Appropriately timed, carefully executed surgery usually has excellent results.

ORBITAL ARTERIOVENOUS MALFORMATIONS

Surgical treatment should be limited to those patients with severe pain, progressive visual loss, intractable glaucoma, or marked exophthalmos with congestion and corneal exposure. Orbital arteriovenous malformations, whose blood supply is derived from the external carotid artery, can be embolized under direct radiographic visualization. Surgical exploration should be designed to isolate and control the blood supply to the lesion. Vascular channels are cauterized or ligated. Controlled hypotensive anesthesia is recommended when operating on vascular tumors.

INFLAMMATORY DISEASES OF THE ORBIT

The original descriptions of "orbital pseudotumor" included many non-neoplastic inflammatory lesions involving various tissues within the orbit. For our purposes, we shall exclude any inflammatory lesion in which a specific etiologic diagnosis can be made, such as infection, Wegener's granulomatosis, and foreign-body reaction. We shall limit our discussion to those lymphoproliferative disorders referred to as idiopathic, inflammatory, orbital pseudotumors. These disorders present a spectrum of orbital disease ranging from spontaneously resolving inflammatory lesions to frankly neoplastic malignant lymphomas. Appropriate management depends not only upon accurate designation of the lesion, but also upon the realization that a given lesion may progress along the histopathologic "spectrum."

The classic signs of orbital pseudotumor include proptosis, motility disturbances, and erythema and swelling of the lids and/or conjunctiva (Fig. 10-4).

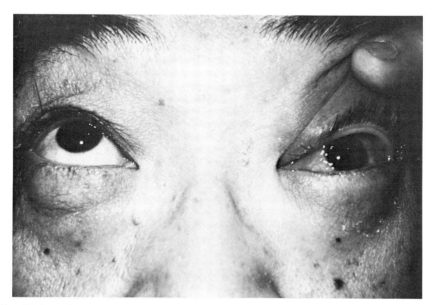

Fig. 10-4. Left-sided ptosis, erythema of the lids, chemosis, and limitation of upward gaze with inflammatory pseudotumor. The lesion was painful and responded to corticosteroid therapy.

Pain is common but is not always present. Some orbital pseudotumors present as a painless space-occupying mass lesion that truly mimics an orbital neoplasm. Onset is most common in middle-aged patients, although all ages may be affected. The inflammatory lesion may present anywhere within the orbit. The globe itself may be involved, especially in adolescents.

Various clinical labels have been attached to orbital pseudotumor, depending on the location of inflammation within the orbit. Inflammation restricted to an extraocular muscle has been termed orbital myositis. Inflammation involving the optic nerve may be referred to as inflammatory perineuritis. Inflammation of the orbital apex and/or cavernous sinus has been referred to as the Tolosa-Hunt syndrome.

A-scan ultrasonography typically reveals a low-reflective lesion. B-scan technique may reveal fluid in Tenon's space, enlargement of the optic nerve shadow, and a mottled pattern to the orbital fat (Fig. 10-5). Findings on CT scan include optic nerve, extraocular muscle, or posterior scleral thickening. A ring of contrast enhancement may be seen around the lacrimal gland. A nonspecific mass lesion simulating an orbital neoplasm can also be seen.

Patients presenting with acute pain, injection, and proptosis are usually

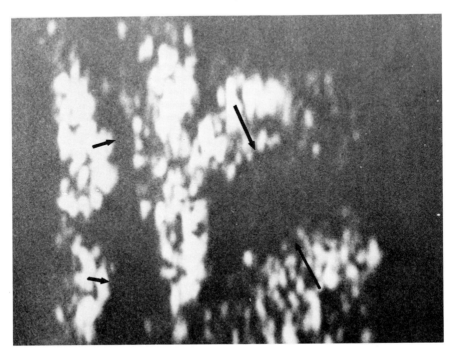

Fig. 10-5. B-scan ultrasound with orbital inflammatory pseudotumor. There is fluid in Tenon's space (short arrows), enlargement of the optic nerve shadow (long arrows), and diffuse mottling of the orbital fat.

found to have idiopathic inflammatory lesions, whereas patients with slowly progressive lesions without pain will often fall into the lymphoma category. It is often impossible, however, to separate inflammatory lesions from malignant lymphomatous masses on the basis of a clinical evaluation. In addition, patients with "inflammatory pseudotumor" may develop signs of systemic lymphoma many years after initial presentation. In contrast, some patients with lesions thought to be characteristic of orbital lymphoma on pathologic examination may never develop systemic lymphoma.

Treatment of patients with presumed inflammatory orbital pseudotumor (based on history, physical, ultrasonography and radiography) is undertaken when there is severe pain, disabling diplopia, or visual loss. Systemic corticosteroid therapy is the treatment of choice in these circumstances. Initial doses of prednisone should range from 40 to 120 mg/day depending on the age and size of the patient. Hospitalization may be preferred for the initiation of high-dose steroids. Consultation with an internist is appropriate. Steroids should be tapered to every-other-day doses as soon as the clinical course will allow. Striking improvement will usually become obvious within 24 to 48 hours. Tapering of corticosteroids must be titrated to the clinical course. If no improvement occurs after five to seven days of steroid therapy in a lesion thought to be inflammatory, biopsy should be done. Patients responding poorly or not at all to steroids should be suspected of having a neoplastic rather than an inflammatory lesion. Alternatively, they may have an inflammatory lesion characterized by a more fibrotic rather than cellular (lymphocytic) architecture. This, however, must be proven by biopsy. Other patients in whom biopsy is indicated are those with an initial spontaneous remission or an initial response to steroids who then suffer a recurrence of orbital involvement.

Biopsy is utilized for clinical–histopathologic correlation. Lymphocytic infiltration with diffusely distributed lymphoblasts and poor steroid responsiveness suggests malignant lymphoma. The histopathologic finding of germinal follicles and spontaneous resolution of clinical findings with corticosteroid therapy suggests benign lymphoid hyperplasia. Eosinophilia is more characteristic of reactive lesions such as inflammatory pseudotumor rather than malignant lymphoma. The presence of significant fibrous infiltration histopathologically may explain a poor clinical response to corticosteroids in otherwise benign lesions.

Immunologic typing of cell-surface immunoglobulins may be of further help in distinguishing malignant lymphoma from benign lymphocytic hyperplasia. Monoclonal patterns of immunoglobulins (all IgG, IgA) suggest malignant lymphoma rather than benign lymphoid hyperplasia. The use of cell-surface markers in determination of malignancy is a relatively new technique that may prove valuable in the future.

Referral to an oncologist and radiotherapist is appropriate when the histopathologic diagnosis of lymphoma is encountered or strongly suspected. Treatment of biopsy-proven orbital lymphoma involves local irradiation. Split doses

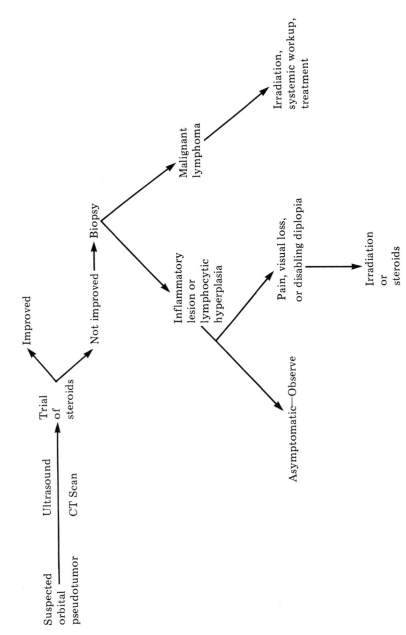

Fig. 10-6. Suspected inflammatory pseudotumor.

of 1500 to 3000 rads have also been used successfully in cases of benign lymphoid hyperplasia. As with thyroid ophthalmopathy, radiation may provide a means of avoiding long-term corticosteroid use. Patients with apparent lymphoid hyperplasia must be observed over the years for evidence of malignant lymphoma. A negative systemic workup in patients with orbital lymphoma does not preclude the potential for systemic involvement years later. Patients with evidence of systemic lymphoma (abnormal bone marrow biopsy, abnormal lymph nodes) may require systemic chemotherapy in addition to local radiation. Surgical staging of the disease is often indicated. Figure 10-6 illustrates a simplified approach to patients clinically thought to have inflammatory orbital pseudotumor.

LACRIMAL GLAND FOSSA LESIONS

Management of the patient with a lacrimal gland fossa mass can be guided by the clinical history, physical examination, and x-ray findings. The major problem is clinical identification of benign mixed lacrimal gland tumors; which should be excised en mass and not biopsied. Other lesions to be considered in the differential diagnosis of lacrimal gland fossa tumors include epithelial malignancies, dacryoadenitis, inflammatory pseudotumor, the spectrum of lymphoproliferative disorders, and dermoid cysts.

Dacryoadenitis presents with a short history (days) and a red, swollen, very tender upper lid. The patient may be febrile and have accompanying enlargement of the preauricular or cervical nodes. Skull x-rays are normal. The white blood cell count will usually be elevated. Appropriate systemic antibiotics will produce resolution. Secondary dacryoadenitis accompanied by characteristic systemic abnormalities may be seen with mumps, infectious mononucleosis, or herpes zoster.

Inflammatory pseudotumor often presents as a painful mass with localized erythema. Motility disturbances may be a concomitant finding. Lymphoma frequently presents as a painless mass. A salmon-colored subconjunctival lesion may be seen. Skull x-rays are usually normal with both pseudotumor and lymphoma.

Dermoid cysts are usually noted in the first decade of life. The patients present with a painless firm mass of the upper eyelid or with progressive proptosis if the lesion is deeply situated in the orbit. Plain skull x-rays will often reveal a sharply defined, scalloped bony defect of the orbital rim in more chronic cases.

Patients with epithelial lacrimal gland tumors can be divided into two groups on clinical grounds. One group is comprised of patients (usually middle-aged) with a history of painless eyelid or superotemporal swelling and proptosis of longer than 12 months. These findings are characteristic of patients with benign mixed lacrimal gland tumors. Radiographic evidence of expansion of the lacrimal fossa is usually present. The second group comprises patients suspected of having lacrimal gland carcinomas. They have a short history, often with pain, and may or may not have abnormal radiographs (Fig. 10-7). These tumors are more common under 35 or over 55 years of age.

The importance of recognizing the first group on clinical grounds cannot be overemphasized. The temptation to biopsy these lesions should be avoided. Incomplete excision of a benign mixed cell tumor may adversely affect the prognosis. Residual tumor cells may lead to tumor recurrence. Although such recurrences are often histologically benign, malignant changes can occur. Malignant recurrences invariably spread beyond the limits of surgical resection.

The initial surgical management of lesions clinically thought to be benign mixed-cell tumors should be total removal of the tumor, lacrimal gland, and adjacent tissues (periorbital, conjunctiva, levator aponeurosis) through a lateral orbitotomy. It is essential to keep the capsule of the tumor intact and to remove overlying periorbita. An anterior orbitotomy often leads to a subtotal or piecemeal removal of the gland and tumor.

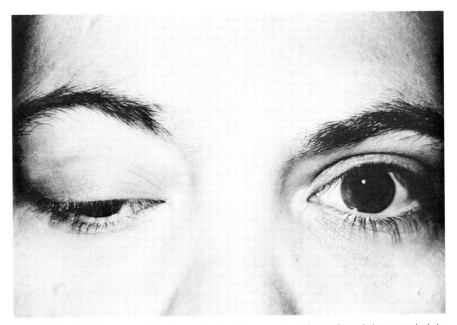

Fig. 10-7. Painful, progressive lacrimal gland fossa mass with ptosis and downward globe displacement on the right side. These symptoms and signs evolved over a two-month period. The patient was found to have adenocystic carcinoma of the lacrimal gland.

Patients with a short history of a lacrimal fossa swelling and associated in-flammatory signs can reasonably be treated with a short course of antibiotics (dacryoadenitis) or corticosteroids (pseudotumor). Resolution within two to three weeks would be the expected course. Unless the mass shows a progressive decrease in size, early incisional biopsy should be done.

Patients with a lacrimal gland mass without inflammatory signs who have a history of shorter than 12 months should also be biopsied. They often complain of pain and show radiologic evidence of invasion of the overlying bone or evidence of calcification within the tumor. An immediate biopsy should be obtained through a trans-septal incision. The extraperiosteal approach does not maintain the integrity of the periosteal barrier, potentially increasing the risk of seeding the extraperiosteal space with malignant cells.

By following this protocol, a definite tissue diagnosis can be reached at an early stage in the clinical evaluation. Such diverse lesions as inflammatory masses, lymphomas, and carcinomas will be accurately identified and the appropriate treatment started.

Patients found to have adenocystic carcinoma and other malignant epithelial neoplasms should be evaluated to determine tumor extent. An attempt at radical resection may be undertaken when the intracranial space has not been violated. The skills of a neurosurgeon and plastic surgeon as well as the ophthalmic surgeon should be united in such a surgical procedure. Surgical resection in these cases should include portions of the lateral and superior orbital walls as well as removal of the lids and orbital contents. Radiotherapy and chemotherapy may be considered in those cases in which spread has occurred beyond even these wide surgical margins. The outlook for these patients is extremely poor.

This approach, summarized in Figure 10-8, diminishes the need for histologic diagnosis by frozen section and permits decisions on extensive surgical removal of a neoplastic lesion to be based on evaluation of permanently fixed microscopic sections. Furthermore, the risks of incisional biopsy of a benign mixed tumor and its subsequent potential recurrences are minimized. This risk cannot be completely eliminated, for occasionally a patient with a benign mixed-cell tumor arising in the palpebral lobe will present with a short history of a slowly enlarging mass similar to a chalazion, and in these circumstances the lesion is invariably approached directly.

No protocol can provide a foolproof solution to the complex decisions facing the surgeon. Nonetheless, this diagnostic approach, based primarily on clinical history and radiologic findings, does provide a logical approach to the problem of lacrimal gland fossa lesions. In part, the dismal prognosis of malignant gland tumors is related to delay in diagnosis, with subsequent spread beyond the limits of surgical excision. An improved survival rate can be achieved by an aggressive attitude towards early biopsy followed by definitive surgery.

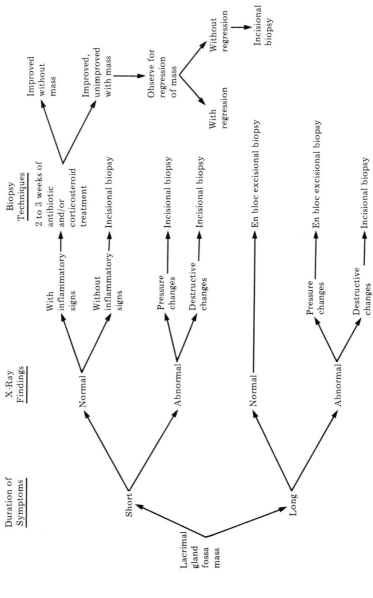

Fig. 10-8. Flowsheet of management of lacrimal gland/fossa masses based on duration of symptoms and radiologic findings. (Short duration less than 12 months; long duration greater than 12 months. Incisional biopsies via transeptal approach. En bloc excisional biopsy done via lateral orbitotomy. Lacrimal gland/fossa mass, with long duration of symptoms and pressure changes on x-ray, is the characteristic presentation of benign mixed cell lacrimal gland tumor.) (Modified from Wright, JE, Stewart, WB, Krohel, GB: Br J Ophthal 63: 600–606, 1979.)

RHABDOMYOSARCOMA

Rhabdomyosarcoma is the most common primary malignant orbital tumor of childhood. The average age of onset is approximately 7.5 years, with 75 percent presenting before 10 years of age. Congenital cases and onset in adulthood, although reported, are uncommon. Males are more often affected than females.

The characteristic presentation is that of rapidly increasing exophthalmos. A subconjunctival or palpebral mass may be present. A superior orbital mass is most commonly reported, although the tumor can occur elsewhere in the orbit (Fig. 10-9). Ptosis is present in nearly one half of the patients secondary to mass effect. Visual loss and pain are less common.

The evaluation of these patients should include plain skull films, hypocycloidal tomography, computerized tomography, and ultrasonography whenever feasible. Hypocycloidal tomography of the sinuses has important prognostic significance. The mortality is approximately four times higher when the sinuses are involved with tumor. The most frequent sites of metastasis are the lungs, lymph nodes, and bone. For this reason, a chest x-ray and bone marrow studies are necessary.

Orbital masses suspicious of rhabdomyosarcoma must be biopsied immediately. An anterior orbitotomy, either trans-septal or trans-conjunctival, is the appropriate surgical approach. An adequate tissue specimen must be obtained.

Throughout the evaluation and especially during management, the ophthalmologist must work hand-in-hand with the oncologist, pediatrician, radiotherapist, and pathologist. Exenteration, which had previously been the treatment of choice, provides only a 30- to 40-percent three-year survival rate. The present role of surgery is to confirm diagnosis by incisional biopsy. Irradiation with chemotherapy, the major treatment modalities at present, can provide up to 90 percent three-year survival in tumors localized to the orbit. Three-year survival is generally equated with cure. Radiation therapy employs up to 6000 rads delivered over a six-week course for local control. A visible response is often seen after

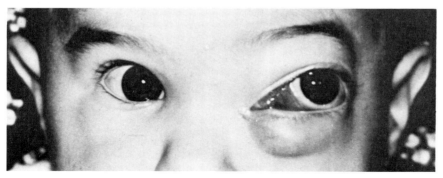

Fig. 10-9. Inferior orbital invasion by rhabdomyosarcoma. This mass is more commonly located in the superior orbit.

delivery of 400 to 600 rads (two to three days), although some patients do not show a response for several weeks. Chemotherapy includes Vincristine, Cyclophosphamide, and Dactinomycin, although protocols are continuously changing.

Patients with metastases should be treated aggressively with focal radiotherapy and lymph node resection when indicated. It is noteworthy that patients with a local recurrence following exenteration may respond favorably to irradiation and chemotherapy. It is satisfying that with recent advances, the survival rate of this highly malignant tumor is increasing without the need for mutilating surgery.

ORBITAL CELLULITIS AND ABSCESS

Orbital cellulitis is a potentially life-threatening infection which must be treated aggressively. Spread to the cavernous sinus may lead to cavernous sinus thrombosis and death. Orbital infections are common, especially in children.

Infections anterior to the orbital septum (preseptal cellulitis) must be differentiated from those posterior to the septum (orbital cellulitis). Preseptal cellulitis presents with lid swelling and erythema. Pain is common. There may be an accompanying fever, leukocytosis, and generalized malaise, especially in children. Motility disturbances, proptosis, and visual loss characterize orbital cellulitis with involvement of structures deep to the orbital septum.

Both preseptal and orbital cellulitis have similar etiologies, which include sinus disease, foreign bodies, spread from contiguous skin infections, and (rarely) hematogenous spread. The organisms most commonly isolated include *Staphylococcus aureus, Streptococcus pyogenes, Escherichia coli,* and *Streptococcus pneumoniae. Hemophilus influenzae* type B is common in children under age 4.

Preseptal cellulitis can usually be treated successfully in adults with an oral penicillinase-resistant antibiotic. This protocol effectively treats the more common streptococcal infections, with coverage for staphylococcus. Children with mild preseptal cellulitis can be treated with oral cefactor that has activity against hemophilus. Children with severe preseptal or orbital cellulitis require treatment with intravenous antibiotics. A penicillinase-resistant agent is employed in combination with either chloramphenicol sodium succinate or ampicillin sodium. The latter choice is dependent on local community sensitivity of *H influenzae* type B infections. Chloramphenicol should not be withheld from a patient with an *H influenzae* infection that is resistant to ampicillin for fear of bone marrow suppression. Orbital cellulitis in adults is treated with a combination of a penicillinase-resistant agent and either penicillin or ampicillin administered parenterally.

Localization of an orbital cellulitis can result in an orbital abscess. Patients who fail to respond rapidly or completely to antibiotic therapy should be suspected of having an orbital abscess. Abscess formation may also occur secondary to spread of infection from adjacent sinuses and dental abscesses. Retained orbital foreign bodies such as wood may lead to an orbital abscess and subsequent osteomyelitis.

Patients with orbital abscess may present in an insidious fashion mimicking an orbital neoplasm. This is especially true of patients who are immunosuppressed. The presence of sinus disease in a debilitated or immunosuppressed patient with proptosis should make one consider the diagnosis of orbital abscess. Similarly, patients with orbital cellulitis who are inadequately treated with oral antibiotics may form an abscess. Pain may be absent in such cases, and the white blood count may be normal. Fever is not always present.

Orbital ultrasound can be useful in differentiating abscess formation from cellulitis. The consolidation of an orbital abscess results in a well-defined lesion with few interfaces, and, therefore, low internal reflectivity. Conventional tomography is valuable in defining the extent of contiguous sinus disease. CT scanning can be useful in defining the location of the abscess, although occasionally only a diffuse inflammatory reaction is noted.

Treatment of orbital abscess requires prompt surgical drainage. A combined otolaryngologic–ophthalmologic approach is usually indicated, as most patients have coexisting sinus infections. Incisions for drainage must be properly placed to decompress the extraperiosteal and intraperiosteal spaces as necessary. Proper drainage must be maintained for several days postoperatively. Stab incisions are often inadequate, especially when the abscess pocket is located posteriorly. Concomitant sinus involvement must also be effectively treated. Unrecognized introduction of foreign bodies should always be suspected, especially in children. Proper surgical exposure is essential in detection and removal of foreign bodies.

An aggressive surgical approach is mandatory when one is dealing with wood and other organic foreign bodies. Incomplete removal of wood splinters can lead to recurrent orbital infections and osteomyelitis of the orbital bones. Reexploration of the orbit may be necessary when orbital infection persists following a foreign body removal. Treatment with antibiotics in such cases without proper surgical drainage may mask the formation of an abscess.

PARANASAL SINUS MUCOCELE

A mucocele results from the continuous or intermittent obstruction of the ostium of the sinus. The retained mucoid material creates pressure that expands the sinus, with thinning and erosion of the bone. The frontal and ethmoidal sinuses are the most frequently involved. With a frontal sinus mucocele, there is often involvement of the adjacent orbital roof, which results in downward displacement of the globe and proptosis (Fig. 4-8). Crepitance may be felt. Radiologically, the scalloped borders of the sinus are lost as the expansion occurs. Treatment consists of surgical drainage with obliteration of the sinus. The mucous membrane lining of the sinus must be completely removed. The sinus is obliterated by packing with adipose tissue acquired from an abdominal incision in an attempt to prevent recurrence. The skills of an otolaryngologist are often required. The posterior bony limits of the sinus must be delineated preoperatively, as neurosurgical assistance may also be needed.

PHYCOMYCOSIS

These serious fungal infections usually occur in diabetics in ketoacidosis. They are also seen in debilitated patients and in patients who are immunosuppressed such as renal transplant recipients. The fungal infection usually originates in the oropharynx or sinuses and spreads to the orbit, with resultant proptosis and motility disturbances. The proptosis is acute, and marked chemosis is often present. Artery occlusion leads to marked tissue necrosis. Complete ophthalmoplegia (frozen globe) usually results. A black eschar is often noted on the palate. Biopsy of necrotic tissue in the nose, mouth, or nasopharynx is necessary to confirm the diagnosis. Vigorous debridement of nonviable tissue is mandatory. Correction of underlying systemic abnormalities such as ketoacidosis is essential if cure is to be achieved. In addition, amphotericin B should be employed, although the prognosis for survival is nonetheless poor.

FIBROUS HISTIOCYTOMA

This tumor of mesenchymal origin is more common in the orbit than originally thought. It occurs most frequently in middle-age, but may occur as early as the second decade. It is a slowly growing, diffusely infiltrating, painless mass. Treatment is surgical, with wide local excision. Recurrences are common. Death can occur secondary to central nervous system invasion. Fortunately, the malignant variant of this tumor is very rare. Fibrous histiocytoma metastatic to the orbit is also rare.

METASTATIC DISEASE IN ADULTS

The primary sites of metastatic tumors to the orbit are the lung in men and the breast in women. Other primary sites include kidney, testicle, prostate, and gastrointestinal tract. As many as one quarter of patients with orbital metastases have an unknown primary at the time of presentation. These patients present a diagnostic challenge that must be shared with an oncologist. In a number of these patients, the primary is never found. Initial findings of metastatic lesions to the orbit are usually decreased visual acuity, diplopia, lid swelling, and ptosis. Conjunctival chemosis and injection may also be present.

Radiotherapy is usually the treatment of choice for local control in patients with orbital metastases and will often afford temporary relief of pain and proptosis. Chemotherapy may also be indicated. Patients with breast carcinoma metastatic to the orbit are often helped by treatment with estrogen receptor antagonists. Occasionally, a well-localized metastasis such as neuroblastoma may be completely excised when no other evidence of systemic tumor is noted.

The surgeon must always obtain adequate tissue for histopathologic review when an orbital metastases is suspected. Electron micropscopy may be helpful in determining the origin of the metastases in undifferentiated carcinomas. With breast carcinomas, tissue for estrogen receptor assay is obtained to help predict the responsiveness of the patient to estrogen receptor antagonist therapy versus other chemotherapy. Other special stains, such as those for acid phosphatase (prostatic carcinoma), may be required by the oncologist and pathologist to help determine the site of the primary tumor.

FIBRO-OSSEOUS TUMORS

Osteoma is a fibro-osseous tumor usually arising in the third or fourth decade of life. The frontal, ethmoidal, and maxillary sinuses are involved more often than the sphenoidal sinuses. Most osteomas are asymptomatic and are noted on skull x-rays taken for other reasons. Facial asymmetry with downward displacement of the globe can occur with large osteomas of the frontal sinus (Fig. 10-10).

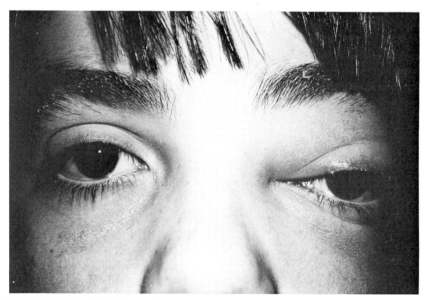

Fig. 10-10. Left-sided frontoethmoidal osteoma with proptosis and inferolateral displacement of the globe.

Osteomas of the sphenoid and ethmoid sinus may infringe on the optic nerve or its blood supply, causing atrophy. In such cases, treatment is surgical and should be undertaken in association with an otolaryngologist.

Fibrous dysplasia may be part of a systemic disease with multiple bone involvement, or it may remain localized to one area of the skeletal system. Isolated craniofacial disease may involve the orbit with resultant proptosis, painless periorbital swelling, and optic atrophy if the optic canals are involved. Marked bony overgrowth may lead to disfigurement. Peak incidence occurs during adolescence.

Surgical decompression of the optic canal by bone removal is indicated when there is stenosis of the optic canal with visual loss and in some cases with severe facial deformities.

DERMOID CYST OF THE ORBIT

The dermoid cyst, usually occurring in the superior temporal or superior nasal aspect of the orbit, is the most frequent benign orbital mass lesion arising in the first two decades, of life.

Dermoid cysts are usually anterior, painless, freely movable, and firm (Fig. 10-11). The mass may extend posteriorly into the middle cranial fossa. There is often

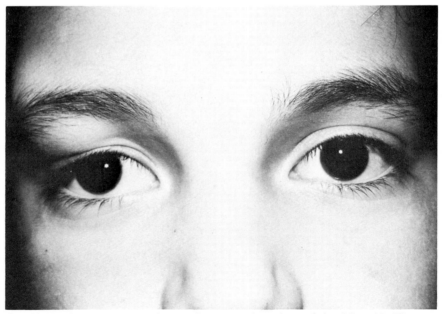

Fig. 10-11. Dermoid cyst in the superior temporal quadrant of the right orbit. The mass was painless and freely movable.

some retrospective evidence (old photographs) in adults suggesting a long-standing process. In difficult cases, the radiographic and ultrasound findings are often diagnostic. Skull x-rays may reveal a smooth cystic defect, usually in the frontal bone. Ultrasound exhibits a smooth, well-defined mass with low internal reflectivity with a "double spike" posteriorly indicative of a cyst wall. CT scanning can demonstrate the extent of the mass. Management, when necessary, is surgery, with delicate dissection of the cyst to avoid rupture. If rupture should occur, adequate irrigation of the cyst contents is necessary to reduce the risk of a significant postoperative inflammatory response.

EOSINOPHILIC GRANULOMA

Eosinophilic granuloma is characterized by isolated bone lesions, often occurring in the frontal or parietal bones, with the outer superotemporal rim most frequently involved. It should be considered apart from the other components of histiocytosis-X (Letterer-Siwe disease and Hand-Schüller-Christian disease), because of its excellent prognosis. Thorough systemic evaluation for additional lesions is essential. Management consists of surgical curettage. Radiation is also reported to be successful, although this modality must be used with caution in children.

OPTIC NERVE GLIOMA

Optic nerve glioma (pilocytic astrocytoma grade 1) will usually present in the first decade of life. Females are more commonly affected than males. Proptosis and loss of vision are the cardinal features of presentation. The proptosis is initially axial, but the eye often becomes displaced downward as the proptosis increases. Optic disc edema or optic atrophy is commonly seen. Strabismus may be present. The clinical course may remain stable over many years or show variable progression. Skull x-rays may reveal an enlarged optic foramen. Suspected involvement of the optic canal can be further verified by basal tomography of the optic canals. CT examination usually reveals thickening of the optic nerve and may demonstrate optic caval and chiasmal abnormalities. The association of optic nerve glioma with neurofibromatosis (Von Recklinghausen's disease) has been well documented. The presence of neurofibromatosis may not be evident when a glioma is initially diagnosed. Stigmata of neurofibromatosis (e.g., café-au-lait spots) should be sought as the child ages, since they may not develop until adolescence. Optic nerve gliomas in association with neurofibromatosis probably represent histologically benign tumors, and tumor proliferation into the subarachnoid space is commonly seen in these patients. In contrast, gliomas in patients without neurofibromatosis do not usually invade the subarachnoid space but rather expand the optic nerve itself. This latter growth pattern is more consistent with a hamartomatous process rather than that of a benign tumor. Despite this pathologic difference, both groups will frequently behave clinically in a similar fashion.

The management of optic nerve glioma remains a controversial subject. No definitive long-term study has yet proven the uncontested superiority of nonsurgical versus surgical management. There is no good evidence that optic nerve gliomas exhibit longitudinal tumor growth. That is, patients with a presumed right optic nerve glioma will probably not experience expansion to the left optic nerve or chiasm. Such a patient, however, may have an unidentified left optic nerve glioma that may expand at a later date simulating tumor spread. On the other hand, optic nerve gliomas definitely expand in a circumferential pattern, either from outward invasion of tumor into the subarachnoid space or by mucoid degeneration within the tumor itself. This circumferential expansion of the orbital portion of the optic nerve can cause cosmetically disfiguring proptosis. Chiasmal involvement may produce hypothalamic disorders, hydrocephalus secondary to ventricular obstruction, and visual loss.

Our clinical approach employs both nonsurgical and surgical therapy depending on the clinical situation. Two major groups of patients can be established based on the radiographic assessment of the optic canals. Patients with suspected gliomas and normal optic canals may be divided into those with useful vision and those with poor vision. Visual function can be assessed with measurement of visual acuity, color vision, pupillary responses, visual field examination, and visual evoked responses. The patient with 20/20 visual acuity may have a severely constricted visual field or an abnormal visual evoked response. Visual-field defects are extremely variable and may include peripheral constriction, depression, or scotoma. Those patients with good visual function may be observed. If visual acuity is markedly compromised (e.g., light perception only) and tumor growth is evident, (i.e., increased proptosis, enlargement of the optic nerve on CT scan) resection of the nerve through a combined craniotomy and intraorbital approach may be indicated. The decision for surgical intervention is influenced by the facts that (1) although rare, meningiomas and other tumors do occur in the first two decades of life and may simulate a glioma, and (2) some optic nerve gliomas demonstrate an aggressive growth pattern. This can lead to compression of intracranial structures, with serious sequelae. If the chiasm is not grossly involved, at surgery the entire optic nerve from chiasm to globe can be removed with hope of "curing" the patient. The globe is preserved. When chiasmal involvement is noted under the operating microscope, the involved nerve is partially resected for tissue diagnosis.

The second major group consists of those patients with abnormal optic canals on radiography. If the optic canal enlargement is unilateral and the visual acuities and visual fields are stable (good or poor vision), the patient may be observed. A craniotomy is recommended if progression is evidenced by deteriora-

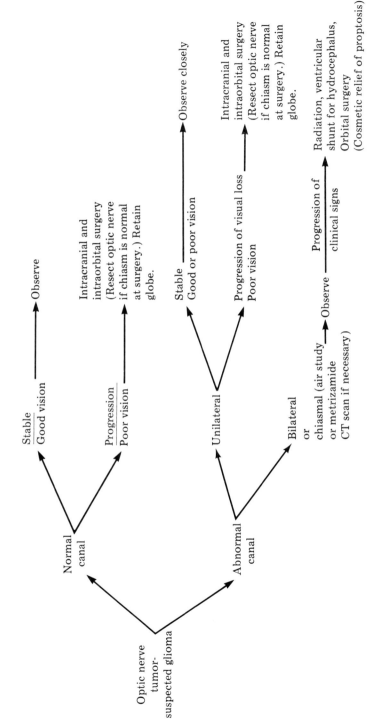

X-ray
Findings

Optic nerve
tumor-
suspected glioma

Normal
canal

Stable
Good vision → Observe

Progression
Poor vision → Intracranial and intraorbital surgery (Resect optic nerve if chiasm is normal at surgery.) Retain globe.

Abnormal
canal

Unilateral

Stable
Good or poor vision → Observe closely

Progression of visual loss
Poor vision → Intracranial and intraorbital surgery (Resect optic nerve if chiasm is normal at surgery.) Retain globe.

Bilateral
or
chiasmal (air study or progression or metrizamide CT scan if necessary) → Observe → Progression of clinical signs → Radiation, ventricular shunt for hydrocephalus, Orbital surgery (Cosmetic relief of proptosis)

Fig. 10-12.   Clinical approach to suspected optic nerve gliomas.

tion of visual function where useful vision is lost. Excision of the affected nerve should be performed if the chiasm is grossly normal at surgery. Careful evaluation of the contralateral eye including visual evoked responses is recommended before submitting the patient to craniotomy. Bilateral abnormalities of optic nerve function, however subtle, indicate chiasmal involvement and mitigate against surgical exploration.

If optic canals are abnormal bilaterally or if the optic chiasm is involved, the tumor is not resectable. Chiasmal involvement may be proven without craniotomy in some patients by high-resolution CT scanning with infusion of metrizamide or pneumoencephalogram. Radiation therapy may affect the course of optic nerve glioma and should be considered when there is chiasmal involvement and relentless, progressive visual loss. The surgical indications in these patients are (1) relief of proptosis by orbital resection of the orbital portion of the optic nerve, and (2) ventricular shunting for relief or hydrocephalus. No patient with useful vision should undergo biopsy or resection of an optic nerve.

This approach to optic nerve gliomas is summarized in Fig. 10-12. Each patient is dealt with individually by assessing the growth pattern of the tumor as objectively as possible. Stable, nonprogressive lesions can be observed, whereas more aggressive gliomas are treated with surgery or irradiation whenever feasible.

NEUROBLASTOMA

In the pediatric population, neuroblastoma is the most common tumor metastatic to the orbit. The majority of patients are younger than 3 years of age, although the tumor has been reported in teenagers. Metastases most frequently involve the zygomatic bone and, therefore, present with a mass in the upper cheek or temple with accompanying proptosis. Ecchymosis of the lids (Racoon sign) is also characteristic. Metastases are bilateral in approximately 50 percent of patients. An abdominal mass should be sought when the diagnosis is suspected. The treatment of metastatic orbital neuroblastoma consists of radiotherapy and chemotherapy. Surgical excision of an orbital neuroblastoma should be considered only when the tumor is an isolated manifestation in the orbit, with no evidence of tumor systemically.

NEUROFIBROMATOSIS

Neurofibromatosis (Von Recklinghausen's disease) is characterized by café au lait spots on the skin and multiple tumors involving both central and peripheral nervous systems. Children with neurofibromatosis have a higher incidence of optic nerve glioma and congenital glaucoma. Neurofibromas of the orbit are either solitary (encapsulated) or plexiform (nonencapsulated). The management of both may involve surgical excision. Complete excision is often impossible with plexiform neurofibromas and reconstructive procedures are often necessary. One must be careful not to sacrifice excessive amounts of involved tissue such as levator muscle, in a vain attempt to achieve a complete excision.

NEURILEMOMA

These peripheral nerve tumors occur in middle age and usually present in the orbit in a fashion similar to cavernous hemangioma. That is, the patient initially presents with slowly progressive, painless proptosis, with visual loss occurring later in the course of the disease. They are only occasionally associated with neurofibromatosis in contrast to optic nerve gliomas and plexiform neurofibromas. Treatment is surgical excision.

MENINGIOMA

Optic Nerve Sheath Meningioma

This tumor characteristically presents in adults with a decrease in visual acuity. Other orbital signs such as proptosis may be subtle or absent. Optic nerve swelling with opticociliary shunt vessels are common findings. CT scan will usually reveal a thickened optic nerve. Basal tomography should be done to rule out invasion of the optic canal. Once satisfied that the tumor is indeed confined to the orbit, the ophthalmologist is then faced with two alternatives. A non-surgical approach may be utilized wherein the patient is maintained under observation. Many patients will retain useful vision for many years. When vision is markedly impaired, the optic nerve can be removed from the back of the globe to the optic foramen via a medial or lateral orbitotomy. The presence of tumor at the posterior aspect of resection indicates a need for neurosurgical exploration of the canal and the chiasm.

An alternative approach involves early biopsy and possible decompression of the optic nerve sheath meningioma. Some patients have an associated optic nerve cyst, which is contiguous with their meningioma. Decompression of this cyst can lead to a partial restoration of visual acuity. In addition, some optic nerve sheath meningiomas will exhibit an exophytic growth pattern. That is, the tumor breaks out through the dura and continues to grow adjacent to the nerve within or without the muscle cone. This portion of the tumor can be removed often with temporary partial return of visual function. It is virtually impossible to completely remove a primary optic nerve sheath meningioma, however, without total loss of vision. Aggressive surgical decompressions, therefore, are aimed at prolonging good visual function rather than curing a patient.

Visual improvement can be anticipated to be temporary, and tumor regrowth is to be expected. Some meningiomas act in a more aggressive manner, with early invasion of the globe and optic canal. These tumors must be approached aggressively and resection effected, even though visual acuity will be lost. A combined neurosurgical and orbital approach is indicated when conventional tomography of the optic canal is abnormal.

Solitary Orbital Meningioma

These are rare tumors that usually cannot be distinguished clinically and radiographically from cavernous hemangiomas or neurilemomas. They probably arise from ectopic meningial cells within the orbit. These tumors behave clinically in a fashion similar to cavernous hemangiomas. The tumor is slow-growing, painless, and usually produces proptosis before or at the same time visual loss is noted. The management of such tumors is essentially the same as that of any progressive localized intraconal mass. That is, complete excision is indicated through a lateral orbitotomy approach.

Sphenoid Ridge Meningioma

These tumors usually present with x-ray evidence of hyperostosis of the greater and/or lesser wings of the sphenoid. Sphenoid wing hyperostosis on x-ray is highly suggestive of meningioma but is not pathognomonic. Osteoblastic metastases to the sphenoid from breast or prostatic carcinoma may produce a similar radiographic appearance.

Visual defects and extraocular muscle palsies are common. Optic atrophy is frequently seen. Management of these tumors consists of craniotomy and resection of the tumor when possible.

Tuberculum-Sella Meningioma

Meningiomas arising from the tuberculum-sella often present in a fashion similar to pituitary adenomas. The patient often presents with bilateral but asymmetrical visual loss. Neurosurgical resection is indicated. These tumors will often grow along the optic nerves and may simulate a primary optic nerve meningioma. In contrast to the sheath meningiomas, these tumors can sometimes be stripped off the optic nerve and removed without loss of vision via a transcranial approach.

Suggested Reading List

GENERAL

Henderson JW: Orbital Tumors. Philadelphia, WB Saunders, 1973

Jones IS, Jakobiec FA: Diseases of the Orbit. Hagerstown, Harper and Row, 1979

Koornneef L: Orbital septa: Anatomy and function. Ophthalmol 86:876, 1979

Lloyd GAS: Radiology of the Orbit. London, WB Saunders, 1975

Lloyd GAS: CT scanning in the diagnosis of orbital disease. Computerized Tomography 3:227, 1979

Ossoinig KC, Blodi FC: Preoperative differential diagnosis of tumors with echography. Part IV. Diagnosis of orbital tumors. In Current Concepts in Ophthalmology. St. Louis, Mosby, 1974, p 313

Reese AB: Tumors of the Eye (3rd ed). New York, Harper and Row, 1976

THYROID OPHTHALMOPATHY

Day RM, Carrol F: Corticosteroids in the treatment of optic nerve involvement associated with thyroid dysfunction. Arch Ophthalmol 79:279, 1968

Donaldson SS, Bagshaw MA, Kriss HP: Supervoltage orbital radiotherapy for Graves ophthalmopathy. J Clin Endocrinol Metab 37:276, 1973

Dixon RS, Anderson RL, Hatt MU: The use of thymoxamine in eyelid retraction. Arch Ophthalmol 97:2147, 1979

Dryden RM, Soll DB: The use of scleral transplantation in cicatricial entropion and eyelid retraction. Trans Am Acad Ophthalmol Otolaryngol 83:669, 1977

Ogura JH, Pratt LL: Transantral decompression for malignant exophthalmos. Otolaryngol Clin North Am 4:193, 1971

Trobe JD, Glaser JS, LaFlamme P: Dysthyroid optic neuropathy: Clinical profile and rationale for management. Arch Ophthalmol 96:1199, 1978

Werner SC: Modification of the classification of the eye changes of Grave's disease. Am J Ophthalmol 83:725, 1977

VASCULAR DISEASES OF THE ORBIT

Flanagan JC: Vacular problems of the orbit. Ophthalmology 86:896, 1979

Haik BG, Jakobiec FA, Ellsworth RM, Jones IS: Capillary hemangioma of the lids and orbit: An analysis of the clinical features and therapeutic results in 101 cases. Ophthalmology 86:760, 1979

Hiles DA, Pilchard WA: Corticosteroid control of neonatal hemangiomas of the orbit and ocular adnexa. Am J Ophthalmol 71:1003, 1971

Jakobiec F, Howard GM, Jones IS, Wolff M: Hemangiopericytoma of the orbit. Am J Ophthalmol 78:816, 1974

Jones IS: Lymphangiomas of the ocular adnexa: An analysis of 62 cases. Trans Am Ophthalmol Soc 57:602, 1959.

Krohel GB, Wright JE: Orbital hemorrhage. Am J Ophthalmol 88:254, 1979

Lloyd GA: Phleboliths in the orbit. Clin Radiol 16:399, 1965

Lloyd GA, Wright JE, Morgan G: Venous malformations in the orbit. Br J Ophthalmol 55:505, 1971

Slusher MM, Lennington BR, Weaver RG, Davis CH: Ophthalmic findings in dural arteriovenous shunts. Ophthalmology 86:720, 1979

Stigmar G, Crawford JS, Ward CM, Thomson HG: Ophthalmic sequelae of infantile hemangiomas of the eyelids and orbit. Am J Ophthalmol 85:806, 1978

Wright JE: Orbital vascular anomalies. Trans Am Acad Ophthalmol Otolaryngol 78:606, 1974

Yee RD, Hepler RS: Congenital hemangiomas of the skin with orbital and subglottic hemangiomas. Am J Ophthalmol 75:876, 1973

INFLAMMATORY DISEASES OF THE ORBIT AND LYMPHOMA

Blodi FC, Gass JDM: Inflammatory pseudotumor of the orbit. Trans Am Acad Ophthalmol Otolaryngol 171:303, 1967

Chavis RM, Garner A, Wright JE: Inflammatory orbital pseudotumor. Arch Ophthalmol 96:1817, 1978

Coop ME: Pseudotumor of the orbit: A clinical and pathological study of 47 cases. Br J Ophthalmol 45:513, 1961

Jakobiec FA, McLean I, Font RL: Clinicopathologic characteristics of orbital lymphoid hyperplasia. Ophthalmology 86:948, 1979

Kennerdell JS, Johnson BL, Deutsch M: Radiation treatment of orbital lymphoid hyperplasia. Ophthalmology 86:942, 1979

Knowles DM II, Jakobiec FA, Halper JP: Immunologic characterization of ocular adnexal lymphoid neoplasms. Am J Ophthalmol 87:603, 1979

Morgan G: Lymphocytic tumor of the orbit. Mod Probl Ophthalmol 14:355, 1975

Morgan G, Harry J: Lymphocytic tumors of indeterminate nature: A five year follow-up of 98 conjunctival and orbital lesions. Br J Ophthalmol 62:381, 1978

Mottow LS, Jakobiec FA: Idiopathic inflammatory orbital pseudotumor in childhood. Arch Ophthalmol 96:1410, 1978

Zimmerman LE, Font RL: Ophthalmologic manifestations of granulocytic sarcoma (myeloid sarcoma or chloroma). Am J Ophthalmol 80:975, 1975

OPTIC NERVE GLIOMA

Glaser JS, Hoyt WF, Corbett J: Visual morbidity with chiasmal glioma: Longterm studies of visual fields in untreated and irradiated cases. Arch Ophthalmol 85:3, 1971

Housepian EM: Surgical treatment of unilateral optic nerve gliomas. J Neurosurg 31:604, 1969

Hoyt WF, Baghdassarian SB: Optic glioma of childhood: Natural history and rationale for conservative management. Br J Ophthalmol 53:793, 1969

Lloyd LA: Gliomas of the optic nerve and chiams in childhood. Trans Am Ophthalmol Soc 72:488, 1973

Miller NR, Iliff WJ, Green WR: Evaluation and management of gliomass of the anterior visual pathways. Brain 97:743, 1974

Spencer WH: Primary neoplasms of the optic nerve and its sheaths. Trans Am Ophthalmol Soc 70:490, 1972

Spencer WH: Diagnostic modalities and natural behavior of optic nerve gliomas. Ophthalmology 86:881, 1979

Stern J, Jakobiec FA, Housepian EM: The architecture of optic nerve gliomas with and without neurofibromatosis. Arch Ophthalmol 98:505, 1980

Taveras JM, Mount LA, Wood EH: The value of radiation therapy in the management of glioma of the optic nerve and chiasm. Radiology 65:518, 1956

Wright JE, McDonald WI, Call NB: Management of optic nerve gliomas. Br J Ophthalmol 64:545, 1980

LACRIMAL FOSSA LESIONS

Ashton NL: Epithelial tumors of the lacrimal gland. Mod Probl Ophthalmol 14:306, 1975

Forrest AW: Epithelial lacrimal gland tumors. Trans Am Acad Ophthaimol Otolaryngol 58:848, 1954

Henderson JW, Neault RW: En block removal of intrinsic neoplasms of the lacrimal gland. Am J Ophthalmol 82:905, 1976

Newton TH: Radiology in lacrimal gland tumors. Radiology 79:598, 1962

Stewart WB, Krohel GB, Wright JE: Lacrimal gland and fossa lesions: An approach to diagnosis and management. Ophthalmology 86:886, 1979

Wright JE, Stewart WB, Krohel GB: Clinical presentation and management of lacrimal gland tumors. Br J Ophthalmol 63:600, 1979

RHABDOMYOSARCOMA

Abramson DH, Ellsworth RM, Tretter P, Wolff JA, Kitchen FD: Treatment of orbital rhabdomyosarcoma. Ophthalmology 86:1330, 1979

Jones IS, Reese AB, Krout J: Orbital rhabdomyosarcoma: An analysis of 62 cases. Trans Am Ophthalmol Soc 63:223, 1965

ORBITAL INFECTIONS

Iliff CE: Mucoceles in the orbit. Arch Ophthalmol 89:392, 1973

Krohel GB, Krauss HR, Christensen RE, Minckler D: Orbital abscess. Arch Ophthalmol 98:274, 1980

Schwartz JN, Donnelly EH, Klintworth GK: Ocular and orbital phycomycosis. Surv Ophthalmol 22:3, 1977

Watters EC, Wallar PH, Hiles DA, Michaels RH: Acute orbital cellulitis. Arch Ophthalmol 94:785, 1976

FIBROUS HISTIOCYTOMA

Jakobiec FA, Howard G, Jones I, Tannenbaum M: Fibrous histiocytomas of the orbit. Am J Ophthalmol 77:333, 1974

Krohel GB, Gregor Z: Fibrous histiocytoma. J Pediatr Ophthalmol Strabismus 17:37, 1980

Stewart WB, Newman NM, Cavender JC, Spencer WH: Fibrous histiocytomas metastatic to the orbit. Arch Ophthalmol 96:871, 1978

MENINGIOMA

Cooling RJ, Wright JE: Arachnoid hyperplasia in optic nerve glioma: Confusion with orbital meningioma. Br J Ophthalmol 63:596, 1979

Karp LA, Zimmerman LE, Bout A, Spencer W: Primary intraorbital mengiomas. Arch Ophthalmol 91:24, 1974

Wright JE: Primary optic nerve meningiomass. Clinical presentation and management. Trans Am Acad Ophthalmol Otolaryngol 83:617, 1977

Wright JE, Call NB, Liaricos S: Primary optic nerve meningioma. Br J Ophthalmol 64:553, 1980

METASTATIC TUMORS

Ashton N, Morgan G: Discrete carcinomatous metastases in the extraocular muscles. Br J Ophthalmol 58:112, 1974

Ferry A, Font R: Carcinoma metastatic to the eye and orbit: I. A clinicopathologic study of 28 cases metastatic to the orbit. Cancer 38:1326, 1976

OPTIC NERVE CYSTS

Krohel GB, Hepler RS: Arachnoidal cyst invading the orbit. Arch Ophthalmol 97:2342, 1979

Miller NR, Green RW: Arachnoid cysts involving a portion of the intraorbital optic nerve. Arch Ophthalmol 93:1117, 1975

Smith JL, Hoyt WF, Newton TH: Optic nerve sheath decompression for relief of chronic monocular choked disc. Am J Ophthalmol 68:633, 1969

ORBITAL SURGERY

Kennerdell JS: Fine needle aspiration biopsy. Arch Ophthalmol 97:1315, 1979

Leone Jr CR: Surgical approaches to the orbit. Ophthalmology 86:930, 1979

Maroon JC, Kennerdell JS: Lateral microsurgical approach to intraorbital tumors. J Neurosurg 44:556, 1976

Norris JL: Orbital endoscopy. Trans Pac Coast Otoophthalmol Soc 59:145, 1978

Wright JE: Orbital surgery, in Silver B (ed): Ophthalmic Plastic Surgery (ed 3). American Academy of Ophthalmol-Otolaryngol Manual. Rochester, 1977, p 213

Wright JE, Stewart WB: Orbital surgery, in Tenzel RR (ed): Ocular Plastic Surgery. International Ophthalmology Clinics. Boston, Little, Brown, 1978, vol 18, no 3, p 149

DERMOID CYST

Cullen JF: Orbital diplopia dermoids. Br J Ophthalmol 58:105, 1974

Jakobiec FA, Bonanno PA, Sigelman J: Conjunctival Adnexal Cysts and Dermoids. Arch Ophthalmol 96:1404, 1978

Pfeiffer ZF, Calhoun J: Dermoids and epidermoids of the orbit. Trans Am Ophthalmol Soc 46:218, 1948

Index